TELL ME
WHEN
IT'S
OVER

Also by Paul A. Offit, M.D.

TELL ME WHEN IT'S OVER

AN INSIDER'S GUIDE to DECIPHERING COVID MYTHS AND NAVIGATING OUR POST-PANDEMIC WORLD

Paul A. Offit, M.D.

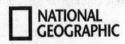

NATIONAL GEOGRAPHIC

Washington, D.C.

Published by National Geographic Partners, LLC
1145 17th Street NW Washington, D.C. 20036

ISBN: 978-1-4262-2366-2

Since 1888, the National Geographic Society has funded more than 14,000 research, conservation, education, and storytelling projects around the world. National Geographic Partners distributes a portion of the funds it receives from your purchase to National Geographic Society to support programs including the conservation of animals and their habitats.

Get closer to National Geographic Explorers and photographers and connect with our global community. Join us today at nationalgeographic.org/joinus

For rights or permissions inquiries, please contact National Geographic Books Subsidiary Rights: bookrights@natgeo.com

Interior design: Nicole Miller Roberts

Printed in the United States of America
23/MP-PCML/1

To Charlotte Moser

In recognition of her relentless dedication
to science and education.
And with appreciation for our long friendship.

CONTENTS

INTRODUCTION

ON DECEMBER 11, 2019, a bat coronavirus made its debut in Wuhan, China. Soon, hundreds of people were hospitalized with pneumonia caused by a virus called SARS-CoV-2. Before the virus left China, more than 4,000 people had died from a disease called Covid. No one was immune. The world was a blank slate.

By January 2020, scientists had isolated the virus and cracked its genetic code. It was now possible to make a vaccine.

In March 2020, the World Health Organization (WHO) declared that the virus sweeping across the globe was officially a pandemic. By that point, 12,000 people had died. In May 2020, after more than 200,000 people in the United States had died from Covid, President Donald Trump announced the creation of Operation Warp Speed, in which the federal government would provide $11 billion to pharmaceutical companies to speed up the development of a vaccine.

In December 2020, after two million people had died from Covid worldwide, the Food and Drug Administration (FDA) authorized vaccines made by Pfizer and Moderna through a streamlined process called Emergency Use Authorization (EUA). Both vaccines contained modified messenger RNA (or mRNA), a novel vaccine technology. Although these mRNA vaccines had been tested in more than 70,000 people—and found to be highly effective—the less stringent EUA approval process, and the breakneck speed with which these vaccines were produced, caused many Americans to worry that corners had been cut—or, worse, that safety guidelines had been ignored. (I am the co-inventor of a rotavirus vaccine, which took 26 years to develop and test. The first Covid vaccines were developed and tested in 11 months.)

In January 2021, after more than 500,000 Americans had died from Covid, Joseph Biden was sworn in as the 46th president of the United States. His administration immediately began mass-producing, mass-distributing, and mass-administering vaccines. Because health systems in the United States weren't geared toward mass-vaccinating adults, this was no easy task. On the day that President Biden was inaugurated, health care workers were vaccinating a million Americans every day. One month later, in February 2021, 1.5 million; in March, 2.5 million; in April, 3.5 million. A remarkable accomplishment.

By June 2023, about 96 percent of the U.S. population, including more than 90 percent of children, had been vaccinated, naturally infected, or both. No longer were hospitals overrun with Covid patients. The original goal of Covid vaccines, which was to prevent serious infections—to keep people out of hospitals, out of intensive care units, and out of morgues—had been reached. Most Americans returned to life as before. In an interview on *60 Minutes,* President Biden said, "The pandemic is over. We still have a problem with Covid. We're still doing a lot of work on it. But the pandemic is over."

Was President Biden right?

One definition of a pandemic is that it changes the way we live, work, and play. An epidemic doesn't. Influenza is a perfect example. Two years before SARS-CoV-2 entered the United States, influenza caused 800,000 hospitalizations and 60,000 deaths. Yearly influenza epidemics don't change the way we live. We don't mask, social distance, isolate, quarantine, restrict travel, shutter schools, close businesses, or test to see if we're infected. If we did, we could dramatically reduce the suffering, hospitalization, and death caused every year by influenza. Indeed, in 2020, when we did all those things to control Covid, influenza virtually disappeared from the United States, as did several other winter respiratory viruses.

We are now at the point where we have accepted the disease and death caused by Covid, as we do with influenza. One thing, however, is certain: SARS-CoV-2 isn't going away. The virus will continue to circulate throughout the world, continue to generate new variants that are more contagious and immune resistant, and continue to cause harm for decades, if not centuries to come—much as has been the case with influenza since the mid-1300s.

PEOPLE ARE NOW throwing away their masks, gathering in indoor settings, attending large sporting events and concerts, using public transportation, going to movies, and getting back to life as normal. We cannot, however, forget that nine million people in this country, because they have weakened immune systems, cannot be vaccinated successfully. Or that about four million babies are born every year in the United States who are susceptible to the virus. Or that tens of millions of Americans are so elderly or have health conditions that are so debilitating that even a mild infection can be life threatening. Also, although Covid vaccines are highly effective at preventing severe disease, they aren't particularly effective at preventing mild disease or eliminating transmission, which will continue to occur even if everyone in the world is vaccinated and even if the virus never creates variants.

How will we live with Covid now while continuing to protect those who are most vulnerable? Do we still need to test and wear masks? Do young children need to be vaccinated? Do Covid vaccine mandates have any place in a post-pandemic world?

THIS BOOK IS ABOUT where we've been and where we're going.

In 2020, I was an attending physician in the Division of Infectious Diseases at the Children's Hospital of Philadelphia when Covid overwhelmed our institution, like many others. I saw children struggling to breathe. I saw parents crying as children were taken to the intensive care unit and mechanically ventilated. And I saw children die. As was the case for so many of us who worked in hospitals, the experience was crushing.

Also in 2020, I was asked by Dr. Francis Collins, head of the National Institutes of Health (NIH), to be part of a group that advised pharmaceutical companies on how to best construct and test Covid vaccines. And I have been a voting member on the FDA's vaccine advisory committee since 2017. Because of my role on these committees, I was often asked to appear on network news programs on CNN, MSNBC, and Fox News, as well as on morning shows on CBS, NBC, and ABC, to explain events that were unfolding in real time. I was frequently quoted in the media, and like many in my position, I felt an enormous responsibility to get things right.

As the pandemic progressed, however, we found that we weren't always right, because our decisions were often based on incomplete information. At times, we would give conflicting recommendations, and as a result, many Americans lost faith in both the institutions and the individuals responsible for guiding us out of this pandemic. In 2022, a Pew Research Center survey found that only 29 percent of adults said they had a great deal of confidence in medical scientists to act in the public's interest. That same year, an NBC News poll found that trust in the Centers for Disease Control and Prevention (CDC) had fallen from 69 percent at the beginning of the pandemic to 44 percent two years later.

In the pages that follow, I invite you behind the scenes to learn as we learned—and will no doubt continue to learn—as SARS-CoV-2 joins the pantheon of other winter respiratory viruses like influenza and respiratory syncytial virus (RSV) that collectively cause hundreds of thousands of hospitalizations and tens of thousands of deaths in the United States every year. We'll trace the rise of Covid conspiracy theories, and how they could endanger our response to future pandemics. And finally, we'll explore how to better protect ourselves and our children against new pathogens. A companion website will provide additional resources and links to the latest science and recommendations.

Our journey will start at the beginning. How and where did this deadly virus originate?

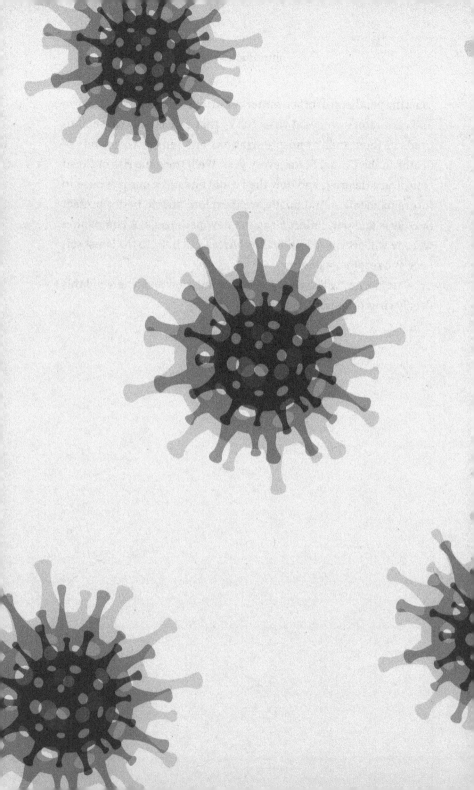

PART I

WHERE
WE WERE

CHAPTER 1

THE ORIGIN OF A NIGHTMARE

- What is SARS-CoV-2?
- Where did SARS-CoV-2 originate?
- Was SARS-CoV-2 created in a laboratory?
- How do we know that SARS-CoV-2 was a product of nature?
- What makes SARS-CoV-2 so dangerous?

WHAT IS SARS-COV-2?

On January 20, 2020, the CDC reported the first case of SARS-CoV-2 infection in the United States. That same day, the agency activated its Emergency Operations Center.

SARS-CoV-2 stands for **s**evere **a**cute **r**espiratory **s**yndrome **co**rona**v**irus, type **2**. When visualized under an electron microscope, coronaviruses look like a crown, which is how they got their name.

What makes SARS-CoV-2 unique?

SARS-CoV-2 isn't the first coronavirus to infect people. Every year, four strains of coronaviruses circulate in the United States. Like SARS-CoV-2, these viruses infect the nose and throat, causing cold-like symptoms; in the most severe cases, they infect the lungs, causing a viral pneumonia. These four coronavirus strains account for about 15 percent of hospital admissions caused by respiratory viruses every winter.

SARS-CoV-2 isn't the first virus to cause a pandemic. Influenza viruses, for example, have caused four pandemics in the last 100 years: specifically, in 1918, 1957, 1968, and most recently in 2009.

SARS-CoV-2 isn't the first coronavirus to cause a pandemic. The first pandemic coronavirus, called SARS-CoV-1, was identified in China in February 2002. The virus spread to 30 countries, infected more than 8,000 people, and killed about 800. By July 2003, the global outbreak was contained; no cases of SARS-CoV-1 have since been reported anywhere in the world.

The second pandemic coronavirus, called MERS (Middle East respiratory syndrome), appeared 10 years later, in June 2012, in Saudi Arabia. The virus spread to 20 countries, infected more than 2,500 people, and killed about 900. Like SARS, MERS is no longer spreading. Both SARS-CoV-1 and MERS viruses originated in bats and then spilled over to infect people.

What makes SARS-CoV-2 uniquely different from all these other viruses is that it has been uniquely devastating. SARS-CoV-1 didn't kill anyone in the United States; neither did MERS. The most recent influenza pandemic of 2009 killed about 12,500 Americans. And the "Great Influenza" pandemic of 1918—the most devastating in U.S. history—killed 675,000 Americans. By April 2023, SARS-CoV-2 had killed more than 1.1 million Americans.

Why has SARS-CoV-2 been so deadly? We'll explore that at the end of this chapter. But first, let's examine where this virus came from. Only with this understanding do we stand a chance of preventing the next pandemic.

WHERE DID SARS-COV-2 ORIGINATE?

Early in the pandemic, the Trump administration made a series of very public mistakes: It was slow to restrict travel from regions where the virus was raging out of control—first Asia, then Europe. It failed to provide enough personal protective equipment to hospitals; nurses were forced to wear garbage bags instead of gowns and bandannas instead of face masks. When ventilators were in short supply, states were left to fend for themselves. Where countries like South Korea, Japan, Canada, and the United Kingdom were quick to provide reliable test kits to define virus hot spots, the United States stumbled out of the gate, initially providing test kits that were inaccurate and had to be recalled. Indeed, President Trump argued that, if anything, Americans were performing too many tests: We were scaring ourselves unnecessarily; the pandemic wasn't really that bad and would likely end by Easter 2020. For his gross mishandling of the early stages of the pandemic, both the press and the public criticized Trump and his administration for its incompetence.

Something had to be done to deflect the blame. Trump settled on not just blaming China for failing to control the virus (referring to SARS-CoV-2 as the "China virus" or "kung flu"), but also on blaming scientists at the Wuhan Institute of Virology for creating it using grants they had received from NIH—grants that had been provided during the Obama administration.

The notion that SARS-CoV-2 either leaked or was deliberately released from a laboratory in Wuhan persisted into the Biden administration. On February 26, 2023, according to a classified intelligence report provided to the White House and key members of Congress, the United States Department of Energy (DOE) concluded that "the Covid pandemic most likely arose from a laboratory leak." No details of how the DOE had reached that conclusion were provided. Two days later, on February 28, Christopher Wray, director of the Federal Bureau of Investigation (FBI), told Fox News that "the FBI has for quite some time now assessed that the origins of the pandemic are most likely a potential lab incident." Again, no details were provided.

The following day, on March 1, 2023, Dr. Marty Makary, a pancreatic surgeon and public health expert, testified before a House select committee. There, he declared that the notion that SARS-CoV-2 originated in a Chinese laboratory was a "no-brainer." Unlike the DOE and the FBI, however, Makary provided details, noting that in 2014 NIH had provided $600,000 to the Wuhan Institute of Virology to study bat coronaviruses. "It's embarrassing [that] we funded the lab," he told the House representatives. He further explained that "the epicenter of the [coronavirus pandemic] is five miles from one of the only high-level virology labs in China. The doctors initially were arrested and forced to sign non-disclosure gag documents. The lab reports have been destroyed; they've not been turned over."

Marty Makary, Christopher Wray, and the DOE all claimed that SARS-CoV-2 had been human-made—something that had never happened before in the history of the world. No pandemic virus has ever been created in a laboratory. If you believe Carl Sagan's statement that "extraordinary claims should be backed by extraordinary evidence," this was an extraordinary claim backed by no direct evidence—only conspiracy and innuendo. "I remain open to any and all evidence supporting a laboratory origin of the pandemic," wrote evolutionary biologist Michael Worobey. "So far, we have no such evidence."

Makary's testimony before a Senate committee wasn't the first time that the "lab leak theory" had been aired before a congressional committee. About two years earlier, on May 11, 2021, before a Senate health subcommittee and the nation, Rand Paul, a Republican senator from Kentucky, grilled Dr. Anthony Fauci, who, as head of the National Institutes of Allergy and Infectious Diseases at NIH, would have been most responsible for providing funds to the Wuhan Institute of Virology. Paul questioned Fauci about how a pandemic virus could have been created in a Wuhan laboratory.

> **Paul:** *Dr. Fauci. We don't know whether the pandemic started in a lab in Wuhan or evolved naturally but we should want to know. Instead, government authorities ... say there is nothing to see here ... To arrive at the truth, the U.S. government should admit that the Wuhan Virology Institute was experimenting to enhance the coronavirus' ability to infect humans ... This gain-of-function research has been funded by the NIH ... Dr. Fauci, do you still support funding the lab in Wuhan?*

What is "gain-of-function" research? And how could such research lead to a devastating worldwide pandemic?

One way to understand gain-of-function is through the prism of the rabies virus. People get rabies when they are bitten by a rabid animal. Once under the skin, the virus travels up the nerves and enters the brain, where it causes delirium, seizures, coma, and invariably death. Rabies is always fatal. Always. It is without question the deadliest infection that humans can contract.

Now, imagine that a scientist engineers a rabies virus so that it is no longer transmitted by the bite of an animal but rather by small droplets from the nose and mouth, like the common cold. This new virus would be highly contagious and uniformly fatal, thereby gaining in function. In the absence of an effective vaccine, it could eliminate humans from the face of Earth.

The good news is that no one has tried to make the rabies virus more contagious. But that doesn't mean it's not possible or that no one would be willing to try. Indeed, in 2012, one experiment so frightened U.S. public health officials that, within two years, federal regulators put laws in place making gain-of-function research illegal.

The experiment took place at the University of Wisconsin–Madison. Researchers took a strain of influenza virus found in birds and altered it so that it could easily grow in ferrets (which, like humans, are mammals). In other words, these researchers had taken a strain of influenza virus that was limited to birds—to which no one in the world was immune—and altered it so that it could cause disease in people. They had created a possible pandemic virus by undertaking gain-of-function research.

After Rand Paul's opening diatribe, Fauci responded quickly and angrily:

> **Fauci:** *Senator Paul, with all due respect, you are entirely and completely incorrect that the NIH has ever done and does now fund gain-of-function research at the Wuhan Institute.*

Rand Paul, a U.S. senator, was one of the first to provide a national platform for the lab leak theory. And he was right about how a pandemic virus could be created during gain-of-function studies. Exactly what studies were performed in the Wuhan Institute of Virology? Was it possible that scientists had created this pandemic virus either intentionally or unintentionally?

WAS SARS-COV-2 CREATED IN A LABORATORY?

In 2016, the lead researcher studying coronaviruses at the Wuhan Institute of Virology was Dr. Zheng-Li Shi (who was often referred to disparagingly by politicians as "the bat lady").

Zheng-Li was studying a coronavirus strain called WIV1 (Wuhan Institute of Virology-1), a bat coronavirus that could grow in monkey cells in the laboratory but didn't cause disease in people. The WIV1 strain bears no resemblance to SARS-CoV-2.

Zheng-Li wanted to see what would happen if she combined WIV1 with each of eight different bat coronaviruses that had been found in caves in and around Wuhan. None of the combination viruses that she created, however, were more dangerous than the strain she had started with (WIV1). Therefore, none of them, like WIV1, could cause disease in people.

So, in a sense, Rand Paul was right: Zheng-Li did perform gain-of-function research. It was possible that she could have created strains of coronaviruses that were more dangerous than WIV1. But that's not what happened. No function was gained.

HOW DO WE KNOW THAT SARS-COV-2 WAS A PRODUCT OF NATURE?

Spillover events from animals to humans are common.

Influenza virus (birds), human immunodeficiency virus (chimps), Ebola virus (bats), mpox (rodents), and the coronaviruses SARS-CoV-1 (bats) and MERS (bats) were all originally animal viruses. Indeed, about 60 percent of human viruses and bacteria originate in animals. (As one pundit noted, the Black Death—caused by the bacterium *Yersinia pestis* [rats]—wasn't created in a medieval biocontainment laboratory.)

Worse, as climate change disrupts animal habitats, many species are being pushed out of their natural homes. Bats, which are victims of these displacements, are a frequent source of these animal-to-human spillover events.

SARS-CoV-2 is the seventh coronavirus known to infect humans and the third in the last 20 years. All these viruses originated in bats. And all originated in sites where animals and people are concentrated in small areas, like so-called wet markets, where different species of live animals are sold. Indeed, SARS-CoV-1 has been traced to two spillover events that occurred in wet markets in Foshan, Guangdong Province, in China in 2002 and again in Guangzhou, Guangdong, in 2003.

As we now know, SARS-CoV-1 wouldn't be the last animal-to-human spillover event in China.

On December 3, 2019, a customer at the Huanan Seafood Wholesale Market, knowing it was illegal to sell certain wild animals, took photographs and videos of the western section of the market, then posted them on Weibo, a Chinese microblogging website. Chinese officials immediately deleted the photographs, but not before a CNN reporter passed them along to scientists in the United States. The photographs showed raccoon dogs and a red fox, both of which are susceptible to coronavirus infections.

One week later, on December 11, 2019, a female vendor in the western section of the market fell ill with Covid. Two of the first three Covid cases had direct contact with the western section of the market. Indeed, more than half of the early cases had direct or indirect exposure to the Huanan market.

Wuhan is a city of 11 million people. A new virus could have arisen in probably 10,000 places, like a school, restaurant, stadium, or shopping mall. Yet in Wuhan, the first cluster of cases was restricted to the western section of the Huanan Seafood Wholesale Market selling live animals susceptible to the virus—exactly where you would expect an animal-to-human spillover event to occur. The estimated chance that this pattern had occurred randomly, and not as a direct result of animals infecting people, is about 1 in 10 million.

Also, Wuhan was a likely place for a pandemic to start. Not because the Wuhan Institute of Virology is there, but because Wuhan is the largest city in central China, home to multiple live animal markets. It's also a major hub for travel and commerce.

Viruses often require heavily populated areas to become established. The Wuhan Institute of Virology wasn't created to start pandemics; it was created to study viruses in a region where a pandemic would most likely start.

In response to the outbreak, the Chinese government closed the market and tested equipment and animals for the presence of SARS-CoV-2. Unfortunately, the Chinese government didn't make the results of those tests available, fueling notions of conspiracy and cover-up. Test results would only become available later, by accident.

Within a few months of the start of the pandemic, the lab leak theory emerged. Proponents of the theory argued that viruses like SARS-CoV-2 aren't found in nature, so the virus must have been created in a lab. But that wasn't true. In 2021, several months after Rand Paul's Senate hearing, researchers at France's Pasteur Institute and the National University of Laos found coronaviruses in bats that had spike proteins virtually identical to the SARS-CoV-2 spike protein. In other words, the spike protein of SARS-CoV-2 *did* exist in nature. It didn't need to be created in a laboratory.

The lab leak theory was further advanced by a popular book titled *Viral: The Search for the Origin of Covid-19,* which gained a lot of media attention. The book was written by Alina Chan, a postdoctoral fellow at the Broad Institute in Cambridge, Massachusetts, and Matthew Ridley, a journalist and author known in part for his skepticism of climate change. Chan and Ridley believed that they had found a smoking gun. They argued that SARS-CoV-2 cannot enter human cells until the spike protein is cut by a protein-cutting enzyme called furin. The authors claimed that the furin cleavage site on the spike protein was weird—something that would only be found in a virus created in a laboratory. However, in May 2023, Chinese investigators identified a bat coronavirus in the Hainan Province that had a furin cleavage site identical to SARS-CoV-2. Again, like the SARS-CoV-2 spike protein, the furin cleavage site was already present in nature.

Scientists who argued against the lab leak theory noted that SARS-CoV-2 wasn't hypertargeted to infect people. The binding of the virus to human cells was loose and promiscuous. Many animals were also infected, including anteaters, baboons, beavers, cats, civets, cougars, deer, dogs, ferrets, gorillas, hamsters, hippopotamuses, hyenas, leopards, lions, lynx, manatees, marmosets, mice, mink, monkeys, otters, pangolins, rabbits, raccoon dogs, tigers, and voles. During the first few years of the pandemic, SARS-CoV-2 became better and better adapted to attaching to human cells and infecting people, evolving to variants like Alpha, Delta, and Omicron. As one scientist quipped, if SARS-CoV-2 had been made in a laboratory, it was made by an underachieving graduate student.

During the Senate hearings, Rand Paul had argued that the Chinese government hadn't found any evidence of SARS-CoV-2 in the animals tested in and around the market. "They've tried to find out if this came from animals, naturally," said Paul. "They checked 80,000 animals to see if it came from the wet market. Not one of them tested positive for Covid-19!" What Paul hadn't realized was that the Chinese *had* found evidence of SARS-CoV-2 in animals in the market. They just hadn't told anyone about it yet.

Finally, in March 2023, a discovery by three prominent researchers—Michael Worobey, an evolutionary biologist at the University of Arizona; Kristian Andersen, a virologist at the Scripps Research Institute in California; and Eddie Holmes, a biologist at the University of Sydney—found the real smoking gun: the one that Chinese officials hadn't initially provided to the scientific community. They noticed that some of the early testing results from the western section of the Huanan Seafood Wholesale Market had appeared briefly, and apparently accidentally, on a website. When the Chinese government realized what had happened, they quickly removed the genetic data. But it was too late.

The evidence was damning. Samples from the Huanan Seafood Wholesale Market first taken in January 2020 showed genetic evidence for SARS-CoV-2 in raccoon dogs that had been sold illegally. In that same area, SARS-CoV-2 was detected in drains, cages, carts, a feather-and-hair remover, a metal cage, and machines that process animals after they have been slaughtered; one stall alone had five positive samples.

One last piece of evidence: It is now clear that two separate lineages of SARS-CoV-2 arose in China at the same time. "There are no tenable scenarios that can explain the presence of both lineages besides two independent zoonotic spillover events," wrote Michael Worobey. "For this to begin as a laboratory accident, one person would have to be infected with lineage B and then immediately go to the Huanan market. Then another person would have to be independently infected with lineage A a week later and also immediately go to Huanan market, each leaving no trace at the laboratory or any other location in a city of 11 million people ... It is virtually certain that the emergence of SARS-CoV-2 was linked to the trade in live wildlife. Anyone who tells you otherwise either doesn't understand the science or doesn't want you to understand it."

On March 11, 2023, Worobey, Andersen, and Holmes appeared on a two-hour 45-minute podcast called *Decoding the Gurus*, where they explained point by point how SARS-CoV-2 traveled from animals to people. This is no longer a scientific controversy.

Despite overwhelming evidence to the contrary, in March 2023, an Economist/YouGov poll found that two-thirds of Americans believed that SARS-CoV-2 was created in a laboratory.

ALTHOUGH RESEARCHERS at the Wuhan Institute of Virology didn't create SARS-CoV-2, the Chinese government was far from blameless. Public health officials in other countries shouldn't have had to depend on a whistleblower in Wuhan to alert the world that a novel virus was spreading unchecked throughout the city, killing hundreds and eventually thousands of people. (Li Wenliang, the 34-year-old ophthalmologist in Wuhan who was the first to warn the world of the coming plague, died from Covid on February 6, 2020. Only later was he was recognized for his heroic actions.)

Worse, Chinese officials consistently claimed that no illegal mammals had been sold at their markets, which was untrue. Four markets in the area sold illegal wildlife, including civets and raccoon dogs, which are known reservoirs for SARS-CoV-2. Indeed, between May 2017 and November 2019, Chinese market vendors sold about 47,000 live animals across 38 species, 31 of which were protected under Chinese law and, therefore, sold illegally. Additionally, the Chinese government was slow to allow scientists from other countries to carefully examine the early series of events in Wuhan, further fueling notions of a conspiracy.

Nevertheless, the lab leak theory will not likely die anytime soon. On April 18, 2023, a 300-page report by Senate Republicans on a health subcommittee stated that "a preponderance of circumstantial evidence [points to] an unintentional research-related incident." Like statements by Marty Makary, Christopher Wray, and the DOE, no specific evidence was provided.

WHAT MAKES SARS-COV-2 SO DANGEROUS?

Although humankind has suffered many pandemic viruses, SARS-CoV-2 was uniquely terrifying for several reasons:

• SARS-CoV-2 is typically spread by people with minimal or no symptoms (that is, asymptomatic). Therefore, anyone, no matter how well they appear, could potentially transmit this deadly virus. In contrast, the first two pandemic coronaviruses, SARS-CoV-1 and MERS, were readily controlled because virtually everyone who was infected got sick. Really sick. So, it was easy to isolate those who were infected and stop the spread of the virus.

• SARS-CoV-2 is constantly creating new strains (variants) that have been more contagious (such as Alpha, Beta, and Delta) or more immune evasive (such as Omicron). People who are fully vaccinated or naturally infected or both can still get mild symptoms with these immune-evasive strains, allowing the virus to continue to spread. To date, no variant virus has arisen that is completely resistant to the protection against serious disease that vaccination or previous infection affords. But it could happen. And more variants are on the way.

• SARS-CoV-2 is particularly deadly for the elderly. More than 80 percent of all Covid deaths have occurred in those over 65 years of age; about 93 percent in those over 55. Indeed, SARS-CoV-2 was known as the "angel of death" in nursing homes, initially accounting for more than 40 percent of all Covid deaths in the United States. For influenza virus, which kills tens of thousands of people every year in the United States, nursing homes account for fewer than 10 percent of deaths.

- Early in the pandemic, SARS-CoV-2 continued to rage during the summer months. No one had expected this. Other respiratory viruses, such as influenza virus, respiratory syncytial virus (RSV), parainfluenza virus, and rhinoviruses (which cause the common cold), among others, typically cause winter diseases. They often disappear during the summer.

- SARS-CoV-2 causes some people to lose their sense of taste or smell for weeks. Scientists have now found that the virus can enter the brain through nerves in the nose.

- SARS-CoV-2 causes prolonged symptoms in some, such as fatigue, memory loss, movement disorders, heart disease, chest pain, "brain fog," and loss of speech—collectively referred to as "long Covid"—with symptoms lasting for months or years.

- SARS-CoV-2 causes a disease called MIS-C, which stands for multisystem inflammatory syndrome in children. This syndrome typically affects children between five and 13 years of age. It starts benignly; children have a mild or asymptomatic infection that resolves quickly. About a month later, after the virus has completely disappeared, children are rushed to the hospital with high fever, pneumonia, and damage to their heart, liver, kidneys, and brain. Children with MIS-C often end up in the intensive care unit and, occasionally, die. By June 2023, more than 9,000 children in the United States had suffered from MIS-C and 76 had died. A similar condition, called MIS-A, occurs in adults.

- SARS-CoV-2 causes inflammation of the lining of blood vessels (vasculitis), which, in addition to causing liver and kidney disease, increases the risk of strokes and heart attacks. Remarkably, SARS-CoV-2 does this without entering the bloodstream. Rather, the virus induces the body's own immune system to destroy cells that line blood vessels. Because every organ in the body has a blood supply, every organ is at risk.

Rand Paul didn't invent the lab leak theory. Exactly one year before Paul's Senate hearing—before vaccines or antivirals or monoclonal antibodies were available to treat or prevent the disease—Covid conspiracy theories were born. The outsize impact of these conspiracy theories on the American public meant that the war against Covid would soon become a war against ourselves.

CHAPTER 2

....

THE LURE OF CONSPIRACY

· When were Covid conspiracy theories born?

· Were any of the original Covid conspiracy theories plausible?

· Why are conspiracy theories so seductive?

WHEN WERE COVID CONSPIRACY THEORIES BORN?

A few months after the start of the pandemic, on May 4, 2020, a slickly made, Hollywood-style film called *Plandemic: The Hidden Agenda Behind Covid-19* aired on several social media outlets. Through brooding music and black-and-white footage, the film introduced the conspiracies that would soon cause people to refuse to wear masks, social distance, test, isolate, quarantine, or receive a Covid vaccine. *Plandemic* was a case study in social engineering.

The movie, which cost only $2,000 to make, centered on two people: Mikki Willis, a little known filmmaker who would later speak at the January 6 insurrection, and Dr. Judy Mikovits, a biochemist.

Willis, a 52-year-old former model and actor, had directed a low-budget indie film called *Shoe Shine Boys*. Before *Plandemic,* he had produced short films on yoga and meditation, a public service announcement on composting, and a documentary about a man who had found a cursed bone in an ancient Maya burial chamber only to be diagnosed months later with bone cancer. (Coincidence? Yes. That's what coincidence is.)

The film opened with an ominous warning: "Now, as the fate of nations hangs in the balance, Mikovits is naming names of those behind the plague of corruption that places all human life in danger." Mikovits then explained that, far from a random act of nature, the Covid pandemic was a coordinated effort by government officials, public health agencies, pharmaceutical executives, evil scientists, billionaires like Bill Gates, and the medical establishment, all of which were willing to open Pandora's box to pad their bank accounts.

The narrator described Judy Mikovits as "one of the most accomplished scientists of her generation [after she] published a blockbuster article in the journal *Science* [that] sent shock waves through the scientific community." Mikovits, however, who would soon become the birth mother of Covid conspiracy theories, wasn't what she appeared to be.

Judy Mikovits began her career in 1988 as a laboratory technician at the National Cancer Institute in Bethesda, Maryland. In 1991, she received her Ph.D. in biochemistry and molecular biology from George Washington University. After leaving Bethesda, Mikovits moved to California, where she served drinks at a yacht club before heading a privately funded research clinic in Reno, Nevada, called the Whittemore Peterson Institute for Neuro-Immune Disease. Scientists at Whittemore were committed to finding the cause of chronic fatigue syndrome, a devastating condition of unknown origin.

In 2009, in a paper published in the prestigious journal *Science*, Mikovits claimed to have found it: People with chronic fatigue syndrome were infected with a mouse retrovirus. Retroviruses are common; most, except for human immunodeficiency virus (HIV), which is the cause of AIDS, are benign. Mikovits believed that she had now discovered another disease caused by a retrovirus. At last, a seeming ray of hope for patients suffering from chronic fatigue syndrome (many of whom began taking potentially dangerous antiviral medications, like those that treat AIDS).

The narrator of *Plandemic* was right to claim that Mikovits's discovery had sent shock waves through the medical community. The shock, however, was short-lived. Two years later, in 2011, the editors of *Science* retracted the paper, stating that "multiple laboratories, including those of the original authors, have failed to reliably detect the mouse retrovirus in chronic fatigue syndrome patients. In addition, there is evidence of poor quality control in several specific experiments." In other words, Judy Mikovits's laboratory had unknowingly contaminated blood samples from patients with chronic fatigue syndrome with a mouse retrovirus. This was a preventable laboratory error and explained why no one else could replicate what she had found. Judy Mikovits's career as a scientist was over. She hasn't published another scientific paper since then.

Mikovits cried foul, refusing to sign the retraction notice in *Science*. To put an end to the controversy, the National Institutes of Health provided $2.3 million to Ian Lipkin, a virologist at Columbia University (who would later serve as chief medical adviser for the movie *Contagion*), to answer the question once and for all. Lipkin's laboratory carefully examined 300 samples of blood from patients with chronic fatigue syndrome in a study that Mikovits agreed would provide "the definitive answer." Lipkin couldn't find what Mikovits had found; mouse retroviruses were not a human pathogen. Nonetheless, Mikovits, who had previously agreed to abide by Ian Lipkin's findings, refused to accept them.

The same year that the editors of *Science* retracted the paper, Annette Whittemore, director of the Whittemore Peterson Institute, fired Judy Mikovits; then Mikovits was arrested on allegations of theft from the institute. The district attorney in Washoe County, Nevada, had charged Mikovits with "possession of stolen property and unlawful taking of computer data, equipment, supplies and other computer-related property." Mikovits fled from Reno, Nevada, to Ventura County, California, where she was arrested as a fugitive and jailed for five days (all criminal charges were eventually dropped).

At this point, Judy Mikovits could have chosen one of two paths. She could have agreed that her laboratory had made a mistake and moved on. She wouldn't have been the first scientist to have published a paper that was wrong and to apologize for the error; in fact, many excellent scientists have done exactly that. Or she could have held fast to the notion that she was right and that everyone else was wrong. Mikovits chose the second path, and a conspiracy theorist was born. This is the person who would later "educate" millions of Americans about Covid and the Covid vaccines.

Plandemic made its debut nine years after Judy Mikovits's *Science* paper had been retracted. By this time, Mikovits had claimed that mouse retroviruses not only caused chronic fatigue syndrome; they also caused autism, lymphoma, and prostate cancer. Mikovits also tried to rewrite history, arguing in *Plandemic* that she "was held in jail with no charges," that the material removed from the Whittemore Peterson Institute had been planted, that a police SWAT team had executed a nighttime raid on her home, and that Anthony Fauci had "threatened her with arrest if she visited the National Institutes of Health to participate in a study to validate her chronic fatigue syndrome research." "I have no idea what she is talking about," said Dr. Fauci.

Four months after SARS-CoV-2 entered the United States and seven months before a vaccine to prevent it became available, *Plandemic* made its debut. Simply put, Judy Mikovits told millions of Americans exactly what they wanted to hear.

WERE ANY OF THE ORIGINAL
COVID CONSPIRACY THEORIES PLAUSIBLE?

Plandemic offered many theories about Covid and Covid vaccines—all of which, as time would tell, were wrong.

Regarding the origin of the virus, Mikovits said, "The virus was manipulated at North Carolina laboratories, Fort Detrick, the U.S. Army Medical Research Institute of Infectious Diseases, and the Wuhan laboratory. It is very clear that it was manipulated. If it was a natural occurrence, it would take up to 800 years to occur." As described in chapter 1, SARS-CoV-2 was a product of nature, not man. And it occurred in the blink of an eye.

Regarding Covid cures, Mikovits said, "the antimalarial drug hydroxychloroquine is the most effective medication to treat Covid-19 ... but they keep it from people." As we'll see in the next chapter, far from keeping it from people, the FDA briefly authorized hydroxychloroquine as a treatment for Covid before realizing that it didn't work and was dangerous.

Regarding masks, Mikovits said, "Wearing the mask literally activates your own virus." SARS-CoV-2 is already activated; it doesn't need a mask to help it become more devastating. On the contrary, because the virus is contained in small droplets in the nose and mouth, masks—which have a pore size much smaller than the droplets—dramatically reduce acquisition and spread of the virus. Nonetheless, Louie Gohmert, a Republican congressman from Texas, feared that he had developed Covid *because* he had worn a mask.

Regarding vaccines as a cause of the Covid pandemic, Mikovits said, "If you've ever had the flu vaccine, you were injected with coronaviruses." Influenza vaccines don't contain coronaviruses. The FDA has strict protocols requiring companies to provide extensive evidence that no extraneous viruses, viral fragments, or viral genes are contained in vaccines. Also, Mikovits contradicted herself when she said that SARS-CoV-2 was created in a lab in Wuhan while at the same time arguing that it had contaminated influenza vaccines and that masks activate it. Which was it? Mikovits's strategy was well worn. Just throw a lot of things up against the wall and hope that something sticks.

Regarding a Covid vaccine, Mikovits said, "There is no vaccine currently on the schedule for any RNA virus that works." This statement alone told you everything you needed to know about Judy Mikovits, who had now become a full-fledged science denialist and anti-vaccine activist.

Mikovits claimed that because SARS-CoV-2 is an RNA virus—which is true—it would be virtually impossible to make a successful vaccine—which isn't true.

Since the 1930s, many successful vaccines against RNA viruses have been made. For example, the yellow fever vaccine virtually eliminated a disease from the United States and Europe that had once killed 10 percent of Philadelphia's population. Before vaccines, polio caused 30,000 cases of paralysis and 1,500 deaths every year in the United States; measles caused 50,000 hospitalizations and 500 deaths; mumps caused 6,000 children to lose their sense of hearing, giving birth to many schools for the deaf; rubella (German measles) infections during pregnancy caused 20,000 children to be born blind and deaf with severe heart defects; and rotavirus caused 75,000 hospitalizations and 60 deaths from dehydration and caused hundreds of deaths every day in the developing world. All these diseases are caused by RNA viruses. And all have been tamed by vaccines.

Regarding the safety of the soon-to-be-released Covid vaccines, Mikovits claimed that companies making the vaccines will "kill millions, as they already have, with their [other] vaccines." By June 2023, more than 13 billion doses of Covid vaccines had been administered in more than 180 countries to 70 percent of the world's population. During that time, SARS-CoV-2 had killed more than seven million people; almost all those deaths occurred in people who had never been vaccinated. In the United States alone, Covid vaccines had saved the lives of at least three million people. Covid has killed millions of people, not the Covid vaccine.

Regarding efforts early in the pandemic to close the beaches, Mikovits said, "Why would you close the beach? You've got healing microbes in the ocean in the salt water. That's insanity." Healing bacteria in the ocean don't exist. Although some viruses (called bacteriophages) can kill bacteria, it doesn't work the other way around. Bacteria don't kill viruses.

Regarding claims of personal freedom, Mikovits said, "If we don't stop this now, we can not only forget our republic and our freedom, but we can forget humanity because we'll be killed by this agenda." Mikovits was firmly in the camp that our country, founded on individual rights and freedoms, should allow people to catch and transmit a potentially fatal virus. Efforts to counter public health measures would soon become a rallying cry for anti-vaccine activists and the political Right.

On the morning of May 5, 2020, about 24 hours after *Plandemic* had debuted on Facebook, YouTube, and Vimeo, a loose, alt-right group called QAnon sent the film to its 25,000 members with the headline, "Exclusive Content, Must Watch." Within hours, 1,700 people had shared the video on their Facebook pages. On the evening of May 5, *Plandemic* appeared on a Facebook page called Reopen Alabama, which included 36,000 members who wanted to lift shelter-in-place orders. Dozens of other Reopen America groups shared the link. More powerful engines of disinformation, such as Collective Action Against Bill Gates, Fall of the Cabal, and Truth Revolution, joined in. Inspired by *Plandemic,* protesters at one anti-vaccine rally shouted, "Arrest Bill Gates."

The next day, on May 6, 2020, *Plandemic* ripped into the mainstream and exploded. Within the week, more than eight million people had seen it on YouTube, Facebook, Twitter (now called X), and Instagram. While *Plandemic* was debuting on Facebook, Taylor Swift announced that she would air her City of Lover concert on television; the cast of *The Office* announced that it would reunite for an 18-minute Zoom wedding; and the Pentagon posted three videos of unexplained "aerial phenomenon." None of these blockbuster cultural events went as viral as *Plandemic,* which apparently was more interesting than alien invasions or Taylor Swift. Celebrities joined in. Comedians Darren Knight and Larry the Cable Guy, mixed martial arts champions Tito Ortiz and Alex Reid, NFL stars, and Instagram influencers all promoted the theories Judy Mikovits spawned.

By the end of May 2020, Mikovits's book, *Plague of Corruption,* which had been published the month before, was #1 on Amazon, beating out Stephenie Meyer's addition to her highly successful Twilight series. "It pays to be a Covid-19 conspiracy theorist," wrote David Gorski, editor of the blog *Science-Based Medicine.* "Before she glommed onto Covid-19, she was a second- or third-string anti-vaccine crank. And now look!"

WHY ARE CONSPIRACY THEORIES SO SEDUCTIVE?

Judy Mikovits and Mikki Willis had carved order out of chaos. While we yearned to understand the source of the virus, Mikovits had provided one (the Wuhan Institute of Virology). While we yearned for a treatment for Covid, Mikovits had offered a readily available drug (hydroxychloroquine). While we yearned to shed our masks,

Mikovits told us why it was OK to throw them away (masks activate the virus). While we yearned to go back to the beaches, Mikovits gave us a reason to open them (healing microbes in the ocean cure Covid). While we yearned for someone to blame, Mikovits gave us villains (Bill Gates, Tony Fauci, the National Institutes of Health, the World Health Organization, and evil scientists in the United States and China).

Years later, researchers would also carve order out of chaos. But the order created by scientific discoveries is much harder earned, much more difficult to understand, and much longer in coming. Conspiracy theories, on the other hand, are easy to understand and only take a few minutes to create and disseminate. Which is why they will never die.

In retrospect, it shouldn't have been surprising that new, deadly viruses give birth to conspiracy theories. When human immunodeficiency virus (HIV) was first identified in 1981, many wondered whether the virus had been created in a laboratory. One of the more outrageous theories at the time was that the Central Intelligence Agency (CIA) had created HIV as a weapon, later testing it in unsuspecting populations in Haiti and Africa, where the experiment had gotten out of control. Indeed, Wangari Maathai, an ecologist in Kenya, who would later win the Nobel Peace Prize, responded to this conspiracy theory at the time saying, "Why has there been so much secrecy about AIDS? That makes me suspicious ... I have always thought that it is important to tell people the truth, but I guess there is some truth that must not be exposed."

In 2010, about 30 years after HIV had entered the United States, scientists showed that a related virus, called simian immunodeficiency virus (SIV), which was first detected in chimps, had evolved into HIV. The evolution of SIV into HIV most likely occurred in Cameroon in the 1930s. Conspiracy theories about lab leaks and the CIA eventually faded away. But it took decades to determine the true origin of the AIDS virus, allowing these theories to flourish.

BY THE MIDDLE OF 2020, thousands of people were dying from Covid every day. The world was desperate for a cure; surely, there must be something available. Something that was being used to treat another disease, but that could also work for this new scourge. Something that was readily available on pharmacy shelves or hospital formularies.

As it turned out, something was available in the early days of the pandemic—something that had been available for more than a hundred years. But it wasn't what everyone was talking about. And it planted the early seeds of distrust in public health agencies—a distrust that would only grow over time.

CHAPTER 3

THE FDA STUMBLES

- Why did the FDA approve a drug to treat Covid that didn't work?
- How do researchers know if a drug works?
- Was anything available in early 2020 that could have saved lives?

When SARS-CoV-2 entered the United States, everyone was susceptible to the ravages of the disease. Everyone. Antivirals wouldn't be available until October 2020, monoclonal antibodies until November 2020, and vaccines until December 2020. Throughout 2020, patients had to suffer with fever, cough, and pneumonia and be taken to intensive care units and hooked up to ventilators, and they sometimes died when little was available to treat or prevent the disease.

The Trump administration was anxious for a magic medicine. Something that was inexpensive and readily available. Something that would put an end to this pandemic.

Enter hydroxychloroquine, a drug to treat malaria.

WHY DID THE FDA APPROVE A DRUG TO TREAT COVID THAT DIDN'T WORK?

Early laboratory studies of hydroxychloroquine as a possible treatment for Covid had been promising. Researchers had shown that chloroquine (a less toxic form of hydroxychloroquine) could treat mice infected with coronaviruses, and that hydroxychloroquine could inhibit coronavirus binding to human cells.

Most of the experimental research, however, was disappointing. For example, hydroxychloroquine didn't cure monkeys infected with SARS-CoV-2. This alone should have been enough to discourage studies in people, especially because hydroxychloroquine was known to cause anemia, seizures, and potentially fatal heart arrhythmias.

The study that gained the most attention was performed by a 68-year-old French researcher named Didier Raoult. In France, Raoult was at one time a star, having won the Grand Prix Inserm, one of France's top scientific prizes. "One of Professor Raoult's abiding characteristics is that he knows he's very good," said Axel Kahn, a geneticist and physician. "But he considers everyone else to be worthless. And he always has." Raoult has called Darwin's theory of evolution "entirely false," believing that Darwin wrote "nothing but inanities." At his home, nestled among a collection of Roman busts, Raoult displays a marble statue of himself.

In March 2020, Raoult headed a small clinical trial of 36 patients with Covid. Twenty patients were treated with hydroxychloroquine; the remaining 16 received standard care. During the following week, all patients were tested for SARS-CoV-2 by polymerase chain reaction (PCR), a test that detects SARS-CoV-2 genes. The treatment, according to Raoult, worked. People treated with hydroxychloroquine had lesser amounts of detectable virus than those who weren't treated. Raoult concluded that hydroxychloroquine had caused "a rapid and effective speeding up of their healing process, and a sharp decrease in the amount of time they remained contagious."

At last, it appeared, something was available to treat Covid.

On March 28, 2020, under intense pressure from the White House, the FDA authorized hydroxychloroquine for the treatment of Covid through a lightning-quick process called Emergency Use

Authorization (EUA). One week later, on April 4, 2020, President Donald Trump ordered the U.S. government to purchase 29 million hydroxychloroquine pills, calling the drug a "game changer." Raoult's findings were called "the study heard 'round the world." Sales of hydroxychloroquine skyrocketed.

Unfortunately, a closer look at Raoult's study revealed that hydroxychloroquine wasn't the miracle drug he had claimed it to be. First, Raoult had only measured the presence of viral genes by PCR, not clinical outcomes, so it was unclear whether the patients who were treated got better faster than those who hadn't been treated. Second, at the start of the study, 26 patients were assigned to the treatment group, but only 20 were reported in the final manuscript. What happened to the other six? As it turned out, one had developed severe nausea; three had required intensive care; one had left the hospital before the treatment could be completed; and one patient had died.

"So, four of the 26 treated patients were actually not recovering at all," said Elisabeth Bik, a scientist who posted a blog about the study. Later, Bik sarcastically mimicked Raoult, saying, "My results always look amazing if I leave out the patients who died."

The degree to which Raoult's study was poorly executed and poorly controlled didn't surprise those who knew him. One prominent French virologist, who chose to speak anonymously for fear of angering Raoult, said that Raoult's reputation among scientists had been "long gone," and that "everybody agrees on the low reliability and reproducibility of most of the papers coming out of his lab." In 2018, two years before the publication of his hydroxychloroquine study, Raoult's lab was stripped of its association with two of France's top public research institutions.

But Didier Raoult wasn't the only person who had cemented President Trump's unshakable belief that hydroxychloroquine was a "game changer."

On July 27, 2020, four months after Raoult had published his study, a group with right-wing ties called America's Frontline Doctors mounted the steps of the Supreme Court in Washington, D.C., to address what they believed was a "massive disinformation campaign" regarding Covid. The 45-minute event, which the Tea Party Patriots organized, was promoted online by the conservative news organization Breitbart as a Supreme Court "press conference," even though it had nothing to do with the Supreme Court. That evening, President Trump shared multiple versions of the video to his 84 million Twitter followers, calling it a "must-watch." The principal speaker, who stood among a group of male physicians in white coats, was a female pediatrician and pastor. "I think they're very respected doctors," said Trump. "There was a woman who was spectacular!"

The "spectacular" woman was Dr. Stella Immanuel. Born in Cameroon in 1965, Immanuel graduated from the College of Medical Sciences at the University of Calabar in neighboring Nigeria. Two years later, in 1992, she moved to the United States, where she practiced medicine out of a strip mall in Houston, Texas. She was also the founder of Fire Power Ministries, a religious organization dedicated to "equipping saints and training warriors for the end times." During the event on the Supreme Court steps, Immanuel described her experience treating patients with Covid. "Nobody needs to get sick," she said. "The virus has a cure—it is called hydroxychloroquine. I have treated over 350 patients and not one death!" According to Immanuel, Americans could now throw away their masks. "Hello! You don't need a mask," she said. "There is a cure."

The day after the event, Facebook removed the video from its platform. But not before incurring the wrath of Stella Immanuel, who warned that Jesus Christ would destroy the social media giant's servers if they didn't restore the video. (Facebook didn't restore the video and never reported an interruption in services.)

This wasn't the first time that Immanuel had made an outrageous claim. During her sermons at Fire Power Ministries, she had preached that alien DNA was used in medical treatments; that scientists were cooking up a vaccine to prevent people from being religious; that cysts, endometriosis, infertility, and miscarriages were caused by women having sex in their dreams with demons and witches ("succubi" and "incubi"); that the government is run by "reptilians" and other aliens ("There are people that are ruling this nation that are not even human," she said); and that a "witch" had concocted a plan to be carried out by the Illuminati to destroy the world using "abortion, gay marriage, and children's toys."

At a White House press conference, Kaitlan Collins, a correspondent for CNN, confronted President Trump. "Mr. President," said Collins, "the woman that you said is a great doctor in that video that you retweeted last night said masks don't work and there is a cure for Covid-19, both of which health experts say is not true. She's also made videos saying that doctors make medicine using DNA from aliens, and that they're trying to create a vaccine to make you immune from becoming religious. It's misinformation." Trump didn't back down, continuing to hold firm to the notion that hydroxychloroquine was America's ticket out of the pandemic. "I thought she was very impressive," answered Trump, "in the sense that, from where she came—I don't know what country she comes from—but she said she's had tremendous success with hundreds of different patients. I thought her voice was an important voice." Trump then abruptly ended the press conference.

HOW DO RESEARCHERS KNOW IF A DRUG WORKS?

The single best way to determine whether a medicine like hydroxychloroquine treats Covid is to perform randomized, controlled clinical trials. Here's how they work: People infected with Covid would be divided into two large groups. One group would receive standard care plus hydroxychloroquine; the other would receive standard care only. For the study to be valid, these two groups of patients must be similar in terms of the severity of their illness, health care–seeking behavior, and other medical problems. Without randomizing subjects to receive the drug or not, the study could be manipulated by the bias of the investigator or the participants. For example, if an investigator was certain that the medicine worked, and wanted to prove it, he or she might be more likely to give the drug to people who were less sick than to those who were sicker. By doing this, the drug would appear to have worked when it really hadn't.

Of interest, Didier Raoult had argued that randomized studies were unethical. "We're not going to tell someone, 'Listen, today's not your lucky day, you're getting the placebo, you're going to be dying.'" (Didier Raoult's statement is the textbook definition of investigator bias.)

In 2020, researchers in the United States, Canada, Brazil, China, Spain, France, South Korea, the Netherlands, and the United Kingdom performed dozens of randomized controlled trials of hydroxychloroquine in tens of thousands of patients. In virtually every study, hydroxychloroquine didn't work to prevent or treat Covid. Three studies, however, put the final nails in the coffin. The names for these studies were RECOVERY, SOLIDARITY, and COALITION.

- RECOVERY: Researchers in the United Kingdom randomly assigned 1,600 patients with Covid to receive hydroxychloroquine plus standard care, and 3,200 to receive standard care alone. Patients who received hydroxychloroquine were more likely to need intensive care, more likely to require mechanical ventilation, and more likely to die than those in the group with standard care only. Hydroxychloroquine not only didn't work, it also worsened outcomes.

• SOLIDARITY: Researchers at more than 400 hospitals in 30 countries randomly assigned 900 patients to receive hydroxychloroquine plus standard care and 900 to receive standard care only. Those who received hydroxychloroquine were more likely to develop severe heart arrhythmias and more likely to die than those who received standard care only. Again, hydroxychloroquine didn't work and was dangerous.

• COALITION: Researchers in Brazil divided 500 patients into three groups. One group received hydroxychloroquine, one received hydroxychloroquine plus Zithromax (an antibiotic that potentiated the effects of hydroxychloroquine), and one received standard care only. Patients receiving hydroxychloroquine with or without Zithromax didn't fare better than those who hadn't received either drug. The only difference was that patients who received hydroxychloroquine were more likely to suffer heart and liver abnormalities. Again, hydroxychloroquine didn't work and was dangerous.

In response to these damning studies, the American Thoracic Society, the European Respiratory Society, the National Institutes of Health, and the Infectious Diseases Society of America strongly recommended against the use of hydroxychloroquine for the treatment of patients with Covid. President Trump, however, remained unconvinced. "All I know is that we've had some tremendous reports," he said. "I've had a lot of people tell me they think it saved their lives." For Trump, it didn't matter what the scientific studies had shown; anecdotes were everything.

On June 15, 2020, only three months after it had authorized the drug, the FDA withdrew its authorization for hydroxychloroquine. Not, however, before millions of people had taken it, some of whom had died as a result. Understandably, Americans were starting to lose faith in the FDA.

After the FDA withdrew its authorization for hydroxychloroquine, Donald Trump and Alex Azar, Trump's handpicked choice to head the Department of Health and Human Services, tried to spin the withdrawal of hydroxychloroquine as something entirely different. "At this point," said Azar, "hydroxychloroquine and chloroquine are just like any other approved drug in the United States. They may be used in hospital; they may be used in out-patients; they may be used at home—all subject to a doctor's prescription." In other words, doctors were free to prescribe a drug that not only didn't work to treat or prevent Covid but was also dangerous. This was a sad day for the Department of Health and Human Services. (When President Trump was admitted to Walter Reed National Military Medical Center with Covid on October 2, 2020, he didn't receive hydroxychloroquine.)

In retrospect, the FDA had failed the American public. When it had authorized hydroxychloroquine for the treatment of Covid, the drug was known to have serious and potentially fatal side effects. Covid was sweeping across the globe; it wouldn't have been hard to find patients willing to participate in studies to see whether the drug worked. Indeed, as it turned out, dozens of studies were performed quickly.

WAS ANYTHING AVAILABLE IN
EARLY 2020 THAT COULD HAVE SAVED LIVES?

In 2020, before monoclonal antibodies, antiviral drugs, or vaccines were authorized, one product was available that could have saved the lives of thousands of Americans who were dying every day from Covid. The product, called convalescent plasma, was made using a technology more than a hundred years old. The country's inability to adequately test and use this product was arguably one of our biggest failures during the early phases of this pandemic.

Convalescent plasma is taken from people who are recovering from an infection. It's been used to treat or prevent infections since the late 1800s. The idea is straightforward: People infected with a virus, assuming they survive, make antibodies against the virus; these antibodies are contained in the liquid (plasma) portion of blood.

In November 2020, monoclonal antibodies became available to treat Covid. But convalescent plasma had always been available.

Convalescent plasma and monoclonal antibodies differ in two important ways. Monoclonal antibodies are directed against one part of one protein of SARS-CoV-2: specifically, the spike protein. Because the spike protein is responsible for attaching the virus to cells, antibodies against the spike protein can prevent infection. Unlike monoclonal antibodies, which bind only one site on the spike protein, the antibodies in convalescent plasma bind several sites on the spike protein, as well as many different sites on the other three SARS-CoV-2 proteins that form the virus.

Convalescent plasma has a long and rich history.

In 1901, Emil von Behring won the first Nobel Prize in Medicine for proving that serum taken from animals injected with diphtheria toxin could treat diphtheria. (Serum is plasma without the clotting factors.) Diphtheria antiserum saved the lives of thousands of children in the early part of the 20th century, and tetanus antiserum was lifesaving during World War I, when tetanus contamination of wounds was common. Antiserum was also used during the 1918 Spanish flu pandemic. Since then, antiserum has been used to treat viral infections such as measles, mumps, chicken pox, hepatitis A, hepatitis B, and Ebola; it's also been used to treat two other pandemic coronavirus diseases, SARS-CoV-1 and MERS. We had, therefore, every reason to believe that plasma obtained from people recovering from Covid, if used early during infection, could successfully treat the disease.

Beginning on April 16, 2020—three months after SARS-CoV-2 had entered the United States—the FDA encouraged blood donations from people who had recovered from Covid. Through the Expanded Access Program, between April and August 2020, before anything else was available to treat or prevent the disease, tens of thousands of people donated their blood to help others—one of the many rays of light that shone during the Covid pandemic.

On Sunday, August 23, 2020, on the eve of the Republican National Convention, the White House held a press conference. Monoclonal antibodies wouldn't be available for three months. Vaccines wouldn't be available for four months. Thousands of Americans were dying every day. Standing at the podium were President Donald Trump, FDA Commissioner Stephen Hahn, and Secretary of the Department of Health and Human Services Alex Azar.

Trump: *I'm pleased to make a truly historic announcement in our battle against the China virus that will save countless lives. The FDA has issued an Emergency Use Authorization ... for a treatment known as convalescent plasma ... It's had an incredible rate of success.*

Azar: *We saw about a 35 percent better survival in patients who benefited most from the treatment, which were patients under 80 who were not on artificial respiration. I just want to emphasize this point because I don't want to gloss over this—this number. We dream in drug development of something like a 35 percent mortality reduction. This is a major advance in the treatment of patients. A major advance!*

Hahn: *Let me just put this in perspective. Many of you know I was a cancer doctor before I became FDA commissioner, and a 35 percent improvement in survival is a pretty substantial clinical benefit. What that means is—and if the data continue to pan out— 100 people who are sick with Covid-19, 35 would have been saved because of the administration of plasma.*

Scientists and physicians were dumbfounded. Thirty-five percent reduction in mortality? What study were Trump, Azar, and Hahn talking about?

The Mayo Clinic study at the center of the August 23, 2020, press conference included more than 2,800 participating hospitals in the United States. Between April and July 2020, as part of the Expanded Access Program, 35,000 patients hospitalized with Covid, many in the intensive care unit, were given plasma from people convalescing from Covid. On August 12, 2020, Mayo Clinic researchers released the results. Researchers had compared patients who had received plasma containing high quantities of SARS-CoV-2 antibodies with those who had received plasma containing lower quantities. They found that the death rate was 8.9 percent in the high-antibody group and 13.7 percent in the low-antibody group. This was good news: People who had received convalescent plasma containing high quantities of antibodies against SARS-CoV-2 were less likely to die from Covid than those given plasma with lower quantities of those antibodies.

When Trump, Azar, and Hahn announced that this study had shown a 35 percent reduction in mortality, however, scientists were angry. One of the senior investigators in the Mayo Clinic study, Dr. Arturo Casadevall, told the *New York Times* that he didn't know where the 35 percent figure had come from.

So, why did Alex Azar and Stephen Hahn say that for every 100 patients with Covid who received plasma therapy, 35 lives would be saved? On Monday evening, August 24, 2020, one day after the news conference, Hahn apologized for his mistake: "I have been criticized for remarks I made Sunday night about the benefits of convalescent plasma," he tweeted. "The criticism is entirely justified. What I should have said better is that the data show a *relative* risk reduction, not an *absolute* risk reduction." The next day, Hahn appeared on *CBS This Morning* and apologized again. But it was too late. "You earn public confidence in small drops," said former FDA commissioner Scott Gottlieb, "and you [lose] it in buckets."

What did Stephen Hahn mean when he said that he had confused relative risk with absolute risk? Here's one way to think about it: If I stand on the sidewalk in front of my house, I have a certain risk of being hit by a car. If I walk across the street in front of my house, I have a much higher *relative* risk of being hit by a car—let's say a thousandfold higher. But the *absolute* risk of my being hit by a car while crossing the street is still very low. (I cross the street in front of my house all the time and have never been hit.)

That was Hahn's mistake. When he said, "What that means is [that of] 100 people who are sick with Covid-19, 35 would have been saved because of the administration of plasma," he had made the false assumption that all people sick with Covid die, which isn't true. Or that all people admitted to the intensive care unit with Covid die, which also isn't true. He should have said that convalescent plasma could save the lives of about 5 of every 100 people sick enough to be admitted to the intensive care unit. Or he could have said that there was a relative risk reduction for severe disease of 35 percent.

The irony of convalescent plasma is that if it had been tested the right way and given early in the illness to those at highest risk, before a patient was hospitalized, it would have been a major lifesaver. As you'll see in chapter 9, antibodies work best early in the disease, when the virus is reproducing itself, and not later in the illness, when the patient is hospitalized.

But at this point in the pandemic, doctors and scientists were still learning about Covid. The Mayo Clinic study tested convalescent plasma only in hospitalized patients—another tragic point on Covid's steep learning curve. (At the end of 2022, circulating variants of SARS-CoV-2 had resisted *all* commercially available monoclonal antibody preparations. For those who couldn't respond to vaccines—such as people who are immune compromised—convalescent plasma was the only way to prevent Covid.)

By the summer of 2020, many Americans no longer trusted anything that Trump, Azar, or Hahn said. The overhyping by Trump (which wasn't surprising), the misrepresentation of the science by the Secretary of Health and Human Services and the FDA commissioner (which was), and the failure of researchers to test convalescent plasma the right way had inadvertently damned the product.

Convalescent plasma usage peaked in the fall of 2020, when more than 40 percent of hospitalized patients received it. By the beginning of 2021, however, fewer than 10 percent of patients were receiving these lifesaving antibodies. The retreat from convalescent plasma was estimated to have caused 29,000 excess deaths between mid-November 2020 and February 2021. However, had it been used the right way—given early in the illness to those at highest risk—hundreds of thousands of lives might have been saved.

DURING HIS ADMINISTRATION, President Trump, like most chief executives, didn't display a deep understanding of science and medicine. The difference between Trump and former presidents, however, was that he was consistently and unabashedly willing to show the public just how little he really did know. ("It ain't what you don't know that gets you into trouble," said Mark Twain. "It's what you know for sure that just ain't so.")

President Trump was confident in his ability to understand and communicate science to the public. During a visit to the CDC in Atlanta in March 2020, a reporter asked him about how the country should prepare for the coming pandemic. "You know, my uncle ... taught at MIT for, I think, like a record number of years. He was a great super genius. Dr. John Trump. I like this stuff. I really get it. People are surprised that I understand it. Every one of these doctors said, 'How do you know so much about this?' Maybe I have a natural ability. Maybe I should have done that instead of running for president."

One month later, on April 24, 2020, Trump suggested that people could treat Covid by injecting themselves with bleach, not understanding that although disinfectants can sterilize surfaces of a variety of germs, they aren't meant to be ingested or injected. "And then I see the disinfectant, where it knocks [the virus] out in a minute. One minute," Trump said at a White House press briefing. Following his statement, the number of accidental poisonings in the United States skyrocketed, forcing Lysol to release a statement pleading with customers not to drink its product.

At the same press conference, as White House staffers watched in horror, Trump soldiered on. He had been told that ultraviolet light, like bleach, could also disable many viruses. But ultraviolet light, which is emitted by the sun, doesn't penetrate beyond the skin. (People don't sunburn their lungs.) Trump had a solution. "So, supposing we hit the body with a tremendous—whether it's ultraviolet or just very powerful light—and I think you said that hasn't been checked, but you're going to test it," he said. "And then I said, supposing you brought the light inside the body, which you can do either through the skin or in some other way, and I think you said you're going to test that, too." Trump was looking at Dr. Deborah Birx, the White House coronavirus response coordinator, who never met Trump's eye. Staring down at her shoes, she appeared to be hoping against hope that the floor would open in front of her, and that this nightmare of a press conference would end.

"For me, it was the craziest and most surreal moment I had ever witnessed in a presidential press conference," said ABC's chief Washington correspondent, Jon Karl. "A few of us actually tried to stop it," said a former White House staffer. Later, at the urging of Mike Lindell, the Trump ally and chief executive of MyPillow, the president agreed that he would "look" at oleandrin, a plant extract, as a treatment for Covid. Lindell had a financial stake in Phoenix Biotechnology, the company that developed oleander-based drugs. He was also a board member.

Given Donald Trump's lack of understanding and disdain for science, his unfortunate promotion of hydroxychloroquine, his mishandling of the convalescent plasma announcement, and his love of bleach, ultraviolet light, and oleander leaves for the treatment of Covid, it is remarkable that his administration was responsible for one of the greatest—if not *the single greatest*—scientific and medical advance of the past one hundred years. And though Donald Trump was quick to embrace treatments that didn't work, were dangerous, or were simply fanciful, he often distanced himself from this one. Even though it was our best way out of the pandemic.

CHAPTER 4

A TICKET OUT

- How long does it take to make a vaccine?
- How were Covid vaccines made so quickly?
- Are vaccines authorized through Emergency Use Authorization (EUA) different than fully licensed vaccines?
- How long does it take to know whether a vaccine causes a serious side effect?
- How do Covid vaccines work?
- Do Covid vaccines cause serious side effects?

The authorization of hydroxychloroquine proved to the American public that the White House could unduly influence the FDA. In August 2020, with the presidential election only three months away, President Trump hinted that a Covid vaccine would be available by October, one month *before* the election—an event he believed would secure his victory. Many public health officials worried that Trump might pressure the FDA to release vaccines before they had been adequately tested.

Would the FDA once again fail to do its job and release a product that hadn't been proven safe and effective? FDA Commissioner Stephen Hahn tried to reassure the public. On August 5, 2020, Hahn wrote an op-ed for the *Washington Post:* "I have been asked repeatedly whether there has been any inappropriate pressure on the FDA to make [vaccine] decisions that are not based on good data and good science. I have repeatedly said that all FDA decisions have been, and will continue to be, based solely on good science and data. The public can count on that commitment." Given that the FDA's decision on hydroxychloroquine hadn't been based on "good science and data," few believed him.

HOW LONG DOES IT TAKE TO MAKE A VACCINE?

On March 23, 1963, at 1:00 a.m., five-year-old Jeryl Lynn Hilleman tiptoed into her father's bedroom and woke him up. "My face hurts," she said. Her father, Maurice Hilleman, was a senior scientist at Merck Research Laboratories. Hilleman examined his daughter, feeling a lump at the angle of her jaw. "Oh, my God," he said. "You've got the mumps." Then Hilleman did something no father does. He got into his car, drove 15 miles to his laboratory, picked up a cotton swab and nutrient broth, went back to the house, gently woke his daughter, stroked the inside of her cheek with the swab, inserted it into the broth, drove back to the lab, put the broth containing Jeryl Lynn's mumps virus in the freezer, and drove home. Four years later, a mumps vaccine was commercially available. Called the Jeryl Lynn strain, it was the fastest vaccine ever made. And it's still used today.

During the past 200 years, beginning with the invention of the smallpox vaccine in the late 1700s, several strategies have been used to make viral vaccines.

After Maurice Hilleman had captured his daughter's natural mumps virus, he weakened it in the laboratory so that when injected into people, it reproduced itself well enough to cause an immune response, but not well enough to cause disease. This is the same strategy that Hilleman used to make the measles, rubella (German measles), and chicken pox vaccines.

Researchers can also take a virus and completely inactivate it with a chemical, which is how the polio and hepatitis A virus vaccines are produced.

Or researchers can use DNA technology to mass-produce just one viral protein, which is how the hepatitis B, human papillomavirus, and one of the influenza vaccines (Flublok) are made. (This is the same technology used to make insulin as well as a wide variety of other medical products.)

Independent of which strategy is chosen, the average length of time it takes to make a vaccine is about 15 years. Why so long?

First, researchers test their vaccines in labratory animals, such as mice or monkeys or ferrets or rats or rabbits, to see whether they work. These are called preclinical or proof-of-concept studies, and usually take many years to complete.

No matter how perfectly a vaccine performs in these preclinical experiments, researchers still must prove that it works in people. (Or, as one famous vaccine researcher said, "Mice lie, and monkeys exaggerate.") So, researchers perform phase 1 studies, in which about a hundred people are divided into several groups. Each group is given a different amount of the vaccine to see whether it elicits an immune response that is likely to be protective. These are called dose-ranging studies. Sometimes researchers find that they must give a larger quantity of the vaccine than they thought was necessary. Sometimes smaller. And sometimes they find that they need to give more than one dose. Or more than two doses. And sometimes they find that they need to have a longer spacing between doses. These studies also take several years to complete.

At this point, researchers believe they know the number of doses, the amount of vaccine in each dose, and the intervals between doses. But they still need to make sure that their vaccine consistently induces an immune response and doesn't have any common serious safety problems. So, they give the vaccine to hundreds of people. These are called phase 2 studies and can be done within a couple of years.

Following the completion of phase 2 studies, researchers are now confident they are on to something. But they haven't proven that the vaccine works in real life, and they haven't shown that it doesn't have uncommon serious side effects. So, they do phase 3 studies. Tens of thousands of people are given the vaccine, and tens of thousands are given a placebo (often salt water). For most adult and pediatric vaccines, these trials take several years to complete.

If the phase 3 studies show that the vaccine is safe and effective, the company then submits data from every phase of development to the FDA for licensure.

HOW WERE COVID VACCINES MADE SO QUICKLY?

SARS-CoV-2 was first isolated in late 2019, and its genome sequenced by January 2020. Eleven months later, two large phase 3 trials of vaccines made by Pfizer and Moderna had been completed. Given that it typically takes about 15 years to make a vaccine, how were these vaccines made in only 11 months?

First, we need to understand some things about SARS-CoV-2.

SARS-CoV-2 consists of four different proteins that surround an RNA genome. ("A virus is a piece of bad news wrapped in a protein coat," said Sir Peter Medawar, a British biologist and author.) Genes are the blueprint that instructs viruses (and cells) on how to reproduce themselves. In the case of SARS-CoV-2, the blueprint is called RNA, which stands for ribonucleic acid. The RNA in SARS-CoV-2 is called messenger RNA (or mRNA), which means that the viral gene can be directly converted into viral proteins.

When researchers were trying to make a vaccine as quickly and efficiently as possible, they figured the best way would be to take the piece of SARS-CoV-2 mRNA that codes for the protein that attaches the virus to cells—the spike protein—and use it to make a vaccine. The antibodies generated by this vaccine would then bind to the spike protein, preventing the virus from attaching to cells and causing an infection. Thus, mRNA vaccines were born. This was the first time in history that a viral gene had been used as a vaccine.

Many Americans—perhaps understandably—feared that mRNA vaccines were too new to be trusted. But in truth, when SARS-CoV-2 first entered the human population in 2019, researchers had been working on mRNA vaccines against other viruses, like the AIDS virus, for about 15 years.

Choosing a vaccine strategy (mRNA) that was fast and efficient wasn't the only reason that the first SARS-CoV-2 vaccines were created so quickly. The other was that the federal government had taken the financial risk out of vaccine development for pharmaceutical companies.

On May 15, 2020, President Donald Trump, in a Rose Garden ceremony at the White House, announced the creation of Operation Warp Speed. To speed up the vaccine process, the federal government announced that it would give $11 billion to vaccine makers. (The term "warp speed" was inspired by the faster-than-light travel used in the popular television series *Star Trek*. Dr. Peter Marks, head of the Center for Biologics Evaluation and Research [CBER] at the FDA, who is a *Star Trek* fan, gave the program its name.) The goal of the program was to produce and deliver 300 million doses of safe and effective Covid vaccines by January 2021. Given that no vaccine against Covid had yet been created, much less tested, that goal was highly ambitious; few thought it was possible.

Operation Warp Speed provided $1 billion to Johnson & Johnson, $1.2 billion to AstraZeneca (a company based in the United Kingdom), $1.5 billion to Moderna, $1.6 billion to Novavax, $2 billion to Pfizer, and $2.1 billion to Sanofi and GlaxoSmithKline. Normally, when you go to the racetrack and bet on a race, you pick one horse to win. The government had bet on several horses to win the same race, refusing to lock in to one company or one vaccine strategy. This approach dramatically increased the government's chances of picking a winner.

Operation Warp Speed turned the timeline for vaccine development on its head. Typically, companies first conduct preclinical studies, then move on to phase 1, then phase 2, then phase 3 trials. If the vaccine works and is safe, companies then mass-produce the vaccine. Companies would never mass-produce a vaccine before knowing that it worked and was safe; it wouldn't be worth the financial risk.

But Operation Warp Speed eliminated that risk. Preclinical studies in mice and monkeys were done over a period of weeks. (Preclinical studies of the rotavirus vaccine we developed at the Children's Hospital of Philadelphia took 10 years to complete.) Phase 1 and 2 studies were combined and involved as few as 20 to 50 participants—instead of the usual hundreds—to determine the right dose. Companies then went directly to phase 3 trials while at the same time mass-producing the vaccine, assuming their studies would show that their vaccine worked and was safe, and if not, millions of doses would be thrown away at no financial risk to the companies. In late 2020, when more than 3,000 Americans were dying from Covid every day, phase 3 studies were completed in three months. (Phase 3 studies for our rotavirus vaccine took four years to complete.)

In May 2020, when President Trump announced the creation of Operation Warp Speed, he said it was, "unlike anything our country has seen since the Manhattan Project." Between 1942 and 1946, in what would later be known as the Manhattan Project, the U.S. government spent $2 billion (the equivalent of $36 billion today) on researching and developing the first nuclear weapons. Trump was right to claim that Operation Warp Speed could be compared to a massive research and development program like the Manhattan Project. But he was wrong to say that "no one has seen anything like this."

In the mid-1950s, 10 years after the Manhattan Project was completed, the March of Dimes, a private philanthropic organization, gave tens of millions of dollars to fund polio vaccine research—especially the work of Dr. Jonas Salk. Salk made his polio vaccine by taking the virus, growing it in monkey kidney cells in his laboratory, purifying it, and then killing it with the chemical formaldehyde. Next, he tested his vaccine in about 700 children in and around Pittsburgh, finding that it was safe and induced high quantities of what he believed would be protective antibodies. The March of Dimes then funded the largest test of a medical product in history. Between 1954 and 1955, 420,000 children were inoculated with Salk's polio vaccine and 200,000 were inoculated with salt water (placebo). After the vaccine had been shown to be safe and effective, the FDA licensed it in two and a half hours.

During the polio vaccine trial, before anyone knew whether it worked or was safe, the March of Dimes funded five companies to mass-produce the vaccine, almost identical to what was later done in Operation Warp Speed. Indeed, the Trump administration's effort to hasten Covid vaccine research and development could reasonably have been called Operation Warp Speed II.

But speed had a price.

Two companies—Eli Lilly and Parke-Davis, both veteran vaccine makers—made the polio vaccine for the large phase 3 trial. The March of Dimes also funded three smaller companies to mass-produce the vaccine before the phase 3 trials had been completed: Wyeth, Pitman-Moore, and Cutter Laboratories. Cutter made the vaccine badly, failing to completely inactivate poliovirus with formaldehyde. Consequently, in 1955, about 120,000 children, primarily in the western and southwestern parts of the United States, were injected with a vaccine made by Cutter Laboratories that contained live, dangerous poliovirus. About 40,000 children suffered short-term paralysis, 164 were permanently paralyzed, and 10 were killed. Called the Cutter incident, it was the worst biological disaster in American history. In addition to giving birth to more stringent vaccine regulation, the Cutter incident served as a cautionary tale as the United States mass-produced Covid vaccines in only a few months and authorized them in only a few weeks.

ARE VACCINES AUTHORIZED THROUGH EMERGENCY USE AUTHORIZATION (EUA) DIFFERENT THAN FULLY LICENSED VACCINES?

In December 2020, when Pfizer's and Moderna's vaccines were first made available to the American public, they weren't *licensed* by the FDA. Rather, they were *authorized* through a less stringent process called Emergency Use Authorization (EUA). Typically, the FDA licenses a vaccine only after reviewing detailed protocols for every step of the manufacturing process. In essence, the FDA licenses not only the vaccine, but also the process by which the vaccine is made, as well as the building in which the vaccine is produced. Once all the data from the phase 3 trials are collected and analyzed, the FDA licensing process typically takes about 10 months. For Covid vaccines, FDA oversight of the processes and buildings occurred while, not after, the final vaccine was being made. As a result, authorization through EUA took about two weeks. In the end, however, there were no differences between licensed vaccines and those approved through EUA. They were the exact same product.

HOW LONG DOES IT TAKE TO KNOW WHETHER A VACCINE CAUSES A SERIOUS SIDE EFFECT?

Typically, to make sure that vaccines don't cause serious side effects, all recipients of experimental vaccines are watched for at least two months after receiving the last dose. This two-month catchment period is critical because vaccines, like all medical products, can cause serious and occasionally fatal problems.

For example, the oral polio vaccine—a live, weakened form of the virus that replaced Jonas Salk's vaccine and was used in the United States from 1962 to 2000—was a rare cause of polio. The yellow fever vaccine is a rare cause of a multi-organ disease that looks like yellow fever. An influenza vaccine used in Europe during the 2009 swine flu pandemic was a rare cause of narcolepsy, a permanent disorder of wakefulness. All these problems occurred within two months of being vaccinated.

For Operation Warp Speed, President Trump had to allow companies to monitor vaccine recipients for at least two months after the last dose. Given the pace of the ongoing trials, the two-month window wouldn't end until the beginning of December, one month *after* the 2020 election.

On September 10, 2020, the Kaiser Family Foundation reported that 62 percent of adults worried that pressure from the White House could cause the FDA to approve a vaccine before it was ready, mimicking the hasty approval of hydroxychloroquine. Amid the confusion, California, Colorado, Connecticut, Michigan, Nevada, New York, Oregon, Washington, West Virginia, and the District of Columbia, fearing that the FDA would bypass its own advisory committee, began to form their own vaccine advisory committees. "The people of this country don't trust this federal government with this vaccine process," said one state governor. Imagine the confusion that would have reigned if some states had approved Covid vaccines and others hadn't. "Do you really want a situation where Texas, Alabama, and Arkansas are making drastically different vaccine policies than New York, California, and Massachusetts?" asked Dr. Saad Omer, an epidemiologist at the Yale Institute for Global Health.

Then the situation worsened.

On October 5, 2020, the *New York Times* reported that top White House officials planned to block new FDA Covid vaccine safety guidelines, which would have delayed vaccine authorization until after the election. The following day, the FDA, to its credit, pushed back, issuing strict guidelines on its website that all vaccine study participants were to be followed *for at least two months after the last dose,* ensuring that vaccine authorization wouldn't occur until after the election. Trump immediately summoned Commissioner Hahn to the White House and—in an invective-laden tirade—insisted that he retreat from his position. But Hahn, to his credit, stood firm.

It is ironic that Donald Trump seemingly picked vaccines to save his presidency. Prior to that, he had shown only contempt for the product. During the Republican presidential debates in 2015, Trump said, "People that work for me, just the other day, two years old, beautiful child, went to have the vaccine and came back a week later, got a tremendous fever, got very, very sick and is now autistic." Trump was referring to the false claim that the measles-mumps-rubella (MMR) vaccine causes autism. At the time, 18 studies in seven countries on three continents had shown that this wasn't true. Trump later invited Andrew Wakefield, the British doctor who had promoted the "MMR causes autism" theory, to one of his inaugural balls. Then he met with Robert F. Kennedy, Jr., who was by that time a prominent anti-vaccine activist, to discuss Kennedy heading a commission on vaccine safety and scientific integrity. Indeed, when Donald Trump was elected president, anti-vaccine activists believed they now had "their man" in the White House. Fortunately, President Trump did nothing to promote the anti-vaccine agenda once elected.

HOW DO COVID VACCINES WORK?

mRNA Vaccines (Pfizer and Moderna)

Researchers at Pfizer and Moderna synthesized the piece of mRNA that coded for the SARS-CoV-2 spike protein and encased it in a small lipid droplet (called a nanoparticle). During the phase 3 trials, Pfizer researchers injected adults with 30 micrograms of this modified viral mRNA and Moderna researchers injected 100 micrograms. (A liquid gram is about one-fifth of a teaspoon. A microgram is one-millionth of a gram. So, this was an extremely small amount of mRNA.) The vaccine was injected into the upper arm, where it entered muscle cells and, for a few days, made SARS-CoV-2 spike protein. Specialized cells of the immune system (called dendritic cells) then took up the protein, broke it down into tiny fragments, and placed it on the surface of the cell. The dendritic cells adorned with spike protein fragments then traveled to the local lymph node under the arm.

Once in the lymph node, these viral protein–decorated immune cells interacted with and activated other cells of the immune system, like B cells (which make antibodies) and T cells (which help B cells make antibodies or kill virus-infected cells). The mRNA vaccines are so powerful that they occasionally cause the lymph nodes under the arm to swell temporarily. Although many vaccines are given as a shot in the arm, no vaccine (apart from the smallpox vaccine) caused lymph node swelling so frequently. A tribute to the ability of mRNA vaccines to stimulate large numbers of immune cells.

Pfizer's phase 3 vaccine trial included about 40,000 adult participants; 20,000 received vaccine and 20,000 received a placebo. Moderna's vaccine trial included 30,000 adult participants; 15,000 received a vaccine and 15,000 received a placebo. Each vaccine was given as a series of two doses, three (Pfizer) or four (Moderna) weeks apart. The phase 3 studies from both mRNA vaccines showed that the vaccines were about 95 percent effective against all manner of symptomatic illness—an amazing result.

(A personal note: I was a voting member of the FDA's vaccine advisory committee in December 2020, when the Pfizer and Moderna vaccines were submitted for authorization. Voting members of the committee are independent advisers with an expertise in infectious diseases, vaccines, and immunology. We are not allowed to hold a position in government, nor are we allowed to have a financial relationship with the pharmaceutical industry. Before the results of the phase 3 studies were available, committee members were informed that we could reasonably recommend authorization of these mRNA vaccines if they were at least 50 percent effective at preventing Covid. A month or so before we saw the results, Dr. Fauci predicted that the vaccines could be as high as 70 percent effective. Everyone was surprised when the vaccines were found to be 95 percent effective. Everyone.)

On December 11, 2020, the FDA authorized Pfizer's vaccine. One week later, the CDC recommended the vaccine for all adults. Pfizer's vaccine then rolled off the shelves and into the arms of Americans. The same sequence of events occurred with Moderna's vaccine one week later.

Viral Vector Vaccines (Johnson & Johnson)

In February 2021, a few months after the approval of Pfizer's and Moderna's vaccines, another Covid vaccine became available, made by Johnson & Johnson (J&J). Researchers at J&J had taken a common cold virus called adenovirus and genetically engineered it so that it couldn't reproduce. It was, in essence, dead virus. Then they inserted the gene that coded for the SARS-CoV-2 spike protein into the adenovirus vector. Once the adenovirus vector was injected into the muscle, the inserted gene would create spike protein mRNA, and the process that followed would mimic that of the mRNA vaccines. The problem with using adenovirus as a Trojan horse to introduce the SARS-CoV-2 spike protein gene into cells is that adenoviruses are common. Most people have already been exposed to these viruses and have antibodies that can neutralize them. To solve this problem, researchers at J&J chose an uncommon human adenovirus called type 26, to which few people have preexisting antibodies.

On February 26, 2021, our FDA vaccine advisory committee met to discuss J&J's vaccine. Unlike the Pfizer and Moderna vaccines, the J&J vaccine was given as a single dose, not a two-dose series like the Pfizer and Moderna vaccines. Like Pfizer, J&J had inoculated 40,000 adults, 20,000 with their vaccine and 20,000 with placebo. Where the Pfizer and Moderna vaccines were about 95 percent effective at preventing symptomatic Covid, J&J's vaccine was 75 percent effective.

What was odd about the J&J submission was that the company had already published a paper in the *New England Journal of Medicine* showing that a second dose of its vaccine clearly increased the quantity of SARS-CoV-2 antibodies. Therefore, it would have made sense to launch J&J's vaccine as a two-dose product as well. Indeed, the company was in the middle of a 30,000-person study with two doses when the FDA met to discuss its one-dose vaccine. Why not wait for the two-dose study to be completed before submitting their vaccine for approval? The company's answer was that one dose still provided a high level of protection against serious illness, and that a single dose might be more acceptable to people who were hard to vaccinate due to travel or homelessness. Additionally, the argument went, the country still didn't have enough vaccines to immunize the entire adult population, so every little bit helped.

A few months later, J&J completed its two-dose vaccine study, finding that two doses were 95 percent effective at preventing Covid, a result almost identical to what had been found with the mRNA vaccines. J&J's vaccine would become a two-dose vaccine. The second dose, however, was not with a J&J vaccine, but rather one of the mRNA vaccines. This unusual dosing schedule was a result of a rare but potentially serious risk with the J&J vaccine that only became apparent after hundreds of thousands of people had been immunized (more on this later).

Protein Vaccine (Novavax)

Vaccines made by Pfizer, Moderna, and J&J employed a similar strategy: Inoculate people with the gene that serves as a blueprint for the SARS-CoV-2 spike protein. People would then use that gene to make the spike protein themselves. Novavax used a more traditional approach. The Novavax vaccines contained the spike protein itself, not the gene that coded for the spike protein. This was the same strategy that had been used to make the hepatitis B vaccine, the human papillomavirus vaccine, and one of the influenza vaccines (Flublok), where people were inoculated with one protein from each of those viruses. The Novavax vaccine also included an adjuvant. (By stimulating the immune system in a variety of ways, adjuvants allow vaccines to be given with lesser amounts of the active ingredient or fewer doses.)

In July 2022, the FDA authorized Novavax's two-dose vaccine for everyone over 18 years of age, and in August 2022, for everyone over 12.

DO COVID VACCINES CAUSE SERIOUS SIDE EFFECTS?

In late 2020 and early 2021, after the FDA had approved the Pfizer, Moderna, and J&J vaccines, and the CDC had recommended them for all adults, everyone held their collective breath. Based on studies of tens of thousands of people, the FDA and CDC had just made recommendations for tens of millions of people. The other shoe had to drop. Historically, it almost always had.

For example, the first biological agent, diphtheria antiserum, killed 13 children in St. Louis when it was found to be contaminated with tetanus; this tragedy caused the U.S. government to pass the Biologics Control Act. The first antibiotic, sulfanilamide, was made palatable for children by suspending it in diethylene glycol, later found to cause kidney failure. More than 100 people died, 34 of whom were children, from ingesting what was called elixir sulfanil-amide. The elixir sulfanilamide disaster led to the birth of the Food, Drug, and Cosmetic Act. Thalidomide, an antinausea drug used for women during pregnancy, was found to cause severe, permanent birth defects in 24,000 babies. The thalidomide tragedy created an amendment to the Food, Drug, and Cosmetic Act to ensure that it would never happen again. ("The history of drug regulation," wrote historian Michael Harris, "is built on tombstones.")

Nonetheless, the tragedies continued. The first chemotherapy—which was administered by one of the world's most famous cancer doctors, Sidney Farber—hastened the deaths of 11 children with leukemia when it was found to contain a growth-promoting instead of a growth-restricting chemical. In 1999, one of the first gene therapies, using a disabled adenovirus like the one used in viral vector Covid vaccines, killed the recipient, a 19-year-old man named Jesse Gelsinger. Again, regulations were put in place to prohibit a repeat of this problem. But it's hard to regulate against the human price often required for medical knowledge; a few years later, 4 of 10 children given a different gene therapy in France developed leukemia.

It was almost inevitable that vaccines soon to be given to hundreds of millions of people would be found to have unexpected, rare, and serious side effects. The only questions were how serious and how rare. After millions of Americans received Covid vaccines, several studies showed an association between mRNA vaccines (that is, Pfizer and Moderna) and myocarditis, which is an inflammation of the heart muscle. The problem occurred primarily within four days of the second dose, mostly in boys and men between 16 and 30 years of age. It was rare, affecting about 1 in 50,000 vaccine recipients. And it was transient, generally resolving within a few days. But it was real. The greatest incidence was in boys 16 to 19 years of age, where the risk was about 1 in 6,600. The risk in children 5 to 11 years of age was 1 in 500,000, about twice as likely as the risk of getting struck by lightning in any given year, which is 1 in 1.2 million.

The other serious health risk, which occurred with the viral vector vaccine (that is, J&J), was severe blood clots, including clots in the brain. The problem occurred mostly in women younger than 40 years of age and was incredibly rare, occurring in about 1 in 200,000 vaccine recipients. Unlike the myocarditis problem, however, brain clots could be fatal, having killed a handful of vaccine recipients by early 2022. Because this was a potentially fatal adverse event, and because the mRNA vaccine problem wasn't nearly as severe, in May 2023, J&J's Covid vaccine was no longer available in the United States.

When Covid vaccines first became available, some people wanted to wait. They argued that FDA officials had authorized vaccines using a lesser standard (EUA) because of the immediacy of the pandemic. Wouldn't it make sense to wait until a few million people had been vaccinated? Indeed, the father of modern vaccines, Maurice Hilleman—a man who had performed the primary research or development on nine of the 14 vaccines given to infants and young children—once said, "I never breathe a sigh of relief until the first three million doses are out there."

A choice not to get a vaccine, however, is not a risk-free choice; it's just a choice to take a different and more serious risk. Covid disease also causes myocarditis. And the risk of myocarditis associated with Covid isn't 1 in 50,000, it's about 1 in 2,000 and far more severe. Covid also causes blood clots. And the risk of blood clots during Covid is also far more common (about 1 in 400) than the 1 in 200,000 risk seen with J&J's vaccine. Again, vaccination was the safer choice.

As is true for many medical decisions, there are no risk-free choices. Probably the greatest risk from vaccines is driving to the doctor's office to get them. About 43,000 people die in car accidents every year: In a U.S. population of 330 million people, that's a yearly risk of 1 in 7,700.

By January 2023, about five billion people—about two-thirds of the world's population—had received at least one dose of a Covid vaccine. Countries with high immunization rates watched as the incidence of hospitalizations and deaths declined. Largely because of Operation Warp Speed, the Trump administration had achieved nothing short of a miracle.

Many assumed that the remarkable success of Covid vaccines would send science denialists and anti-vaccine activists to the sidelines. That the public would no longer tolerate misinformation, fearmongering, and conspiracy theories. That everyone would finally appreciate vaccines to be the lifesaving products they were. Unfortunately, it didn't work out that way.

IN THE YEARS FOLLOWING the entrance of SARS-CoV-2 into the United States, millions of Americans would embrace the ideas launched in *Plandemic,* throwing away their masks, gathering in large crowds, and refusing vaccines. By April 2023, an estimated 330,000 people in the United States had died unnecessarily. But Judy Mikovits and Mikki Willis didn't spread these dangerous ideas by themselves. They needed the help of others to convince millions of Americans to act against their own interests and the interests of their children. Next, we'll learn who these people were, who funded them, and how and why they were so successful.

CHAPTER 5

THE MISINFORMATION BUSINESS

- What single event triggered the birth of the anti-vaccine movement?
- Why did the anti-vaccine movement tilt to the Right during the Covid pandemic?
- Who funds the anti-vaccine movement?
- Who are the leaders of the anti-vaccine movement, and are Covid vaccines as harmful as they claim?

WHAT SINGLE EVENT TRIGGERED THE BIRTH OF THE ANTI-VACCINE MOVEMENT?

On April 19, 1982, a local NBC affiliate in Washington, D.C., aired a one-hour documentary titled *DPT: Vaccine Roulette*. The film featured several children with withered arms and legs, seizing, drooling, staring vacantly up at the sky. The culprit, as described by the fraught parents interviewed for the program, was the whooping cough (pertussis) vaccine. Our children were fine, they pleaded, and now look.

Believing that the film explained some of her son's developmental problems, Barbara Loe Fisher, a marketing executive, launched a parent advocacy group called Dissatisfied Parents Together (DPT). Portions of *Vaccine Roulette* aired on news programs across the country. Now, finally, parents had an explanation for their children's epilepsy or developmental delays or attention deficit disorder or hyperactivity or other neurological problems. Congressional hearings, lawsuits, and mass protests followed. In response to a flood of crushing litigation, vaccine makers left the business. Before the airing of *DPT: Vaccine Roulette*, 18 companies made vaccines for U.S. children; within a few years, only four remained. The rout was on.

Soon after the airing of *Vaccine Roulette*, Dissatisfied Parents Together changed its name to the National Vaccine Information Center (NVIC). For reporters, Barbara Loe Fisher and NVIC became the one-stop shop for parents' views on vaccines. It wasn't long before the anti-vaccine movement moved into the mainstream; Fisher was asked to be a voting member on the CDC's Advisory Committee on Immunization Practices (ACIP) and later the FDA's vaccine advisory committee.

During the next few years, studies showed that children who had received the pertussis vaccine weren't at greater risk for neurological problems. Then, in 2010, 30 years after *Vaccine Roulette* aired, an Australian researcher named Sam Berkovic found that the children featured on the program had suffered from a genetic defect called Dravet syndrome, which causes an abnormal transport of sodium in and out of brain cells. All children with Dravet syndrome suffer neurological problems in the first year of life, regardless of whether they have received a pertussis vaccine.

To their credit, public health agencies and academic centers had taken parents' concerns about the pertussis vaccine seriously, performing dozens of studies showing that the vaccine wasn't to blame. But it didn't matter. Vaccines, once considered lifesaving products, were now claimed to cause a variety of chronic disorders.

In 1987, when a vaccine to prevent *Haemophilus influenzae* type b (Hib), a common cause of meningitis, pneumonia, and bloodstream infections, was first made available in the United States, Barbara Loe Fisher appeared on ABC's *World News Tonight* with

Peter Jennings to warn the public that it caused diabetes. In 2000, when a vaccine to prevent pneumococcus, another significant cause of meningitis, pneumonia, and bloodstream infections, was introduced, Fisher appeared on ABC News to claim that it caused seizures. In 2006, when a vaccine to prevent human papillomavirus, the only known cause of cervical cancer, was introduced, Fisher again appeared on national television claiming that it caused chronic fatigue syndrome. During the next few years, dozens of studies showed that all these claims were incorrect. But the anti-vaccine movement only grew stronger.

Nothing, however, fed America's distrust of vaccines more than an event that occurred in England 16 years after the release of *Vaccine Roulette*. On February 28, 1998, Andrew Wakefield, a British surgeon, and his co-authors published a paper in the *Lancet*—one of the oldest, most respected medical journals in the world—claiming that the combination measles-mumps-rubella (MMR) vaccine caused autism. The report included eight children who had developed autism within one month of receiving the vaccine.

Newspapers carried Wakefield's claim as fact, even though he hadn't proven that children who had received the MMR vaccine were more likely to develop autism than those who hadn't received it. All Wakefield had proven was that the MMR vaccine didn't prevent autism. (The MMR vaccine is designed to prevent measles, mumps, and rubella, not everything else that occurs in life.) Nonetheless, thousands of parents in the United Kingdom chose not to give their children the MMR vaccine; hundreds were hospitalized with measles, and four died from the disease.

Andrew Wakefield became an international hero. At last, someone had boldly stepped forward to speak truth to power, to take on the pharmaceutical companies and their well-paid lobbyists. During the next few years, 18 studies involving hundreds of thousands of children and costing tens of millions of dollars showed that children who had received the MMR vaccine were not at greater risk of autism than those who hadn't received it.

Andrew Wakefield refused to believe these studies. While parents of children with autism cheered him on, and with the strength of a religious conviction, Wakefield continued to promote his false claims. He appeared on morning and evening news shows. On the television program *60 Minutes*, Ed Bradley praised Wakefield for his efforts. Wakefield testified in front of congressional committees. Attractive, well spoken, earnest, and with a British accent, Wakefield was convincing because he was convinced, scientific studies be damned.

Thousands of parents in the United States chose not to give their children the MMR vaccine. As a result, measles—a disease that had been eliminated from the United States by 2000—came back. Hundreds of children were hospitalized. By the early 2000s, propelled by the charisma of Andrew Wakefield and the marketing skills of Barbara Loe Fisher and NVIC, the anti-vaccine movement was flying high.

Enter Brian Deer, a British investigative journalist.

Deer pulled back the curtain on Andrew Wakefield. On February 22, 2004, six years after Wakefield's *Lancet* paper had appeared, Deer published the first in a series of articles in the *Sunday Times* of London. He found that Wakefield had misrepresented the stories of the children in his *Lancet* publication, at least one of whom had developed autism *before,* not after, receiving the vaccine. Also, unbeknownst to his co-authors, Wakefield had submitted a patent on a "safer" measles vaccine. Deer also found that Wakefield had received the equivalent of about $800,000 from the Legal Services Commission; five of the eight children in the *Lancet* paper were suing pharmaceutical companies.

When these revelations came to public attention, the editor of the *Lancet* retracted Wakefield's paper and England's General Medical Council struck him off the medical register. No longer able to practice medicine in England, Wakefield fled to the United States, where his star continued to fall. His last appearance on mainstream television was in 2011 on *Anderson Cooper 360*. Wakefield had appeared on Cooper's show hoping to promote his book, *Callous Disregard: Autism and Vaccines—The Truth Behind a Tragedy*. By this time, however, many studies had shown that Wakefield was wrong. "But, sir," said Cooper. "If your study is a lie, your book is a lie." Wakefield countered by saying that he was the victim of a witch hunt by pharmaceutical companies that had conspired against him.

From that moment on, Andrew Wakefield was limited to appearances on programs like *The Alex Jones Show* and to talks in venues like the Conspira-Sea cruise, where he could commiserate with fellow conspiracy theorists. As his star plummeted, the strength and credibility of the anti-vaccine movement plummeted with him. For the anti-vaccine movement, the situation would only get worse.

In 2014, an epidemic of measles swept across the United States. It started in a community near the Disneyland theme park in Southern California, where parents had chosen not to give their children the MMR vaccine. At the time, California, like all states, had vaccine mandates for school entry. And, like all but two states (Mississippi and West Virginia), it had a vaccine opt-out—specifically, a philosophical exemption, which was granted liberally.

Richard Pan, a state senator from Sacramento and a pediatrician, was concerned that his state had been the epicenter of a measles outbreak. So, on February 19, 2015, Pan introduced Senate Bill 277 to eliminate the philosophical vaccine exemption. If it passed, California parents could only avoid vaccinating their children by homeschooling them or by obtaining a medical exemption from their doctors (which, sadly, several doctors were willing to provide for a fee—even for children who didn't qualify).

Because hearings were open to the public, anti-vaccine activists showed up in droves, violently protesting the bill. Richard Pan was the focus of their ire. One sign read, "PAN-icking over measles!? Get real! Where is the PAN-ic over 1 in 68 with autism?! Vote NO on SB 277!!" Activists spray-painted Pan's house and physically threatened him. Senator Pan had to hire a security guard to follow him around, later obtaining a restraining order against one activist.

During the hearings on Senate Bill 277, anti-vaccine activists resorted to the playbook they had created 35 years earlier after *DPT: Vaccine Roulette,* claiming that vaccines caused autism, diabetes, epilepsy, attention deficit disorder, hyperactivity, birth defects, and all manner of chronic childhood illnesses. By 2015, however, when Richard Pan introduced his bill, many studies had shown that none of these claims were correct. Scientific studies had caught up to the fears. The mainstream media wasn't listening anymore. In response, anti-vaccine activists grew louder, meaner, and more violent—all in a futile attempt to get the press and the public to hear their cries. Senate Bill 277 passed. On June 30, 2015, Governor Jerry Brown signed it into law.

Only a few years before the Covid pandemic, anti-vaccine activism had been marginalized, largely ignored by the public and mainstream press. That would soon change. During the Covid pandemic, activists found the secret sauce that allowed them to reap a bonanza of funding and popular support. Joshua Coleman, the anti-vaccine activist who had been the subject of Richard Pan's restraining order, went on Facebook Live to make an all-too-accurate prediction of what was to come. "This is the one time in human history where every single human being across this country is going to have an interest in vaccination and vaccines," he said. "So, it's time for us to educate." "Educate," in the upside-down parlance of the anti-vaccine movement, meant "misinform."

WHY DID THE ANTI-VACCINE MOVEMENT TILT TO THE RIGHT DURING THE COVID PANDEMIC?

In 2015, soon after the humiliating defeat for anti-vaccine activists in the California legislature, Renée DiResta, a researcher at Stanford, noticed "an evolution in messaging" in Twitter posts from anti-vaccine activists. No longer were activists focusing on false claims about vaccine safety. Rather, the focus now was on "medical freedoms," which activists believed would resonate better with legislators.

This change in messaging was put to the test when Jason Villalba, a well-meaning Republican legislator in Texas, filed a bill in Austin almost identical to California's SB277. As noted by Rekha Lakshmanan, the director of a pro-vaccine advocacy group called the Immunization Partnership, Villalba had unwittingly kicked a hornet's nest. "All of a sudden we saw a kind of new generation of the anti-vaccine movement in Texas emerge," said Lakshmanan. Villalba's bill never got to a vote. Instead, it inspired the creation of a group called Texans for Vaccine Choice to lobby against this and similar legislation. The "freedom" message united anti-vaccine groups, linking them to the Tea Party movement and eventually the Freedom Caucus. Republicans like Jason Villalba could no longer risk opposing "freedom of choice" for vaccines.

During the five years before SARS-CoV-2 entered the United States, heartened by the events in Texas, anti-vaccine activists built a vast network of political action committees across the country. Medical decisions are private, they argued. Our bodies are autonomous. Vaccines are a matter of individual liberties and freedom of choice. The government has no right to tell us what we can or can't put into our bodies or the bodies of our children. These decisions are ours to make, not the government's.

Public health had morphed into private decisions, the public be damned.

Covid restrictions strengthened the marriage between medical freedoms and the Republican Right, giving birth to the ReAwaken America Tour, which held events throughout 2021 and 2022 in Florida, Michigan, Oklahoma, California, Colorado, and Texas (where it was backed by QAnon advocates). Attendees were charged $250 for general admission and $500 for VIP tickets. The tour featured Trump loyalists such as Michael Flynn, who pleaded guilty to lying to the FBI; Roger Stone, who was convicted of lying to Congress and witness tampering; and Mike Lindell (the MyPillow and oleander leaves guy). It also featured a group called America's Frontline Doctors, which included doctors such as Stella Immanuel, who had convinced Trump to embrace hydroxychloroquine; Scott Jensen, who was among those who won Politifact's "Lie of the Year" award for spreading misleading information about Covid and Covid vaccines; and Simone Gold, who claimed that Covid vaccines didn't work, that the pandemic was not a public health emergency, and that FDA-approved vaccines were actually "an experimental biological agent deceptively named a vaccine."

Conservatives who attended the ReAwaken America Tour now had a reason to avoid vaccination. By July 2021, 86 percent of registered Democrats but only 54 percent of Republicans had been vaccinated. By the end of October 2021, 25 of every 100,000 people in counties that heavily supported Donald Trump had died from Covid. In counties that heavily supported Biden, the rates were as low as 0.4 deaths per 100,000—a 60-fold difference. People started calling the Covid pandemic "Red Covid."

Events in Tennessee showed how dangerously far the anti-vaccine, anti-science, anti–public health message had gone. In mid-July 2021, Dr. Michelle Fiscus, Tennessee's medical director in charge of vaccinations, was fired after a Republican representative named

Scott Cepicky argued that her efforts to vaccinate the public—which included allowing mature minors to make their own medical decisions—were "reprehensible." The state then suspended vaccine education, promotion, and outreach for *all* vaccines, not just the Covid vaccines. "I think it's been this insidious growth of their influence on susceptible legislators," lamented Fiscus, "especially in southern states where they have taken the 'medical freedom ... angle' to its illogical end." Fiscus and her family left Tennessee. She is currently the chief medical officer for the Rockville, Maryland–based Association of Immunization Managers.

The Republican assault on vaccines isn't likely to end any time soon. On December 13, 2022, Florida governor Ron DeSantis filed a successful petition with the Florida Supreme Court to launch an investigation into "any and all wrongdoing in Florida with respect to Covid-19 vaccines." Before a presidential run, Ron DeSantis had made Covid vaccine denialism his calling card. In 2023, anti-vaccine activism reached its illogical end when Republican lawmakers in North Dakota, Idaho, and Florida introduced legislation making the administration of mRNA vaccines a crime.

How did this happen?

It's easy to point to cultural and political shifts. Or to the fact that we are a more cynical, more litigious, more distrusting society. Though all this is true, the explanation might be more frightening. Two researchers at Duke University, in a paper titled "Of Pandemics, Politics, and Personality," took a closer look at the personality profile of the anti-vaccine activist.

The liberal-conservative divide in vaccine uptake is contrary to conservatives' moral value system, which includes respect for tradition, authority, the sanctity of institutions, and the law. Indeed, most conservatives aren't anti-vaccine activists, so it seems unfair to paint them with a broad brush.

In reviewing eight studies involving thousands of participants, the Duke researchers found that only a small percentage of people were likely to create, promote, and disseminate misinformation about vaccines. Participants in these studies were assessed for a variety of personality traits. One trait stood apart from the rest: the "need for chaos," which was defined as "a drive to disrupt and destroy the existing order of established institutions to secure the superiority of one's own group over others." Investigators noted that this mindset most likely comes into play when people "feel they are being marginalized and rejected by the broader cultural environment."

Which brings us to the days before Joseph Biden was to be sworn in as the 46th president of the United States.

On January 6, 2021, about 2,500 people broke into the United States Capitol seeking to overturn the results of the presidential election by disrupting a joint session of Congress. The Capitol was locked down and lawmakers and staff were evacuated as rioters broke windows, overturned desks, and attacked law enforcement officers, 140 of whom were wounded. Five people died during the insurrection and four officers who responded to the attack later died by suicide. More than 30 members of anti-government, right-wing, extremist groups, including the Oath Keepers, Proud Boys, and Three Percenters, were charged with conspiracy for planning the attack. Two leaders of the Oath Keepers, Stewart Rhodes and Kelly Meggs, were later convicted of seditious conspiracy and sentenced to 18 and 12 years in jail, respectively. When the dust settled, more than 1,000 insurrectionists were charged with a crime and more than 250 were jailed.

Anti-vaccine activists Charlene and Ty Bollinger were also there, supporting a rally just a few blocks from the Ellipse, where Donald Trump's words to a crowd of supporters on January 6, 2021, would result in an accusation during his second impeachment of inciting the mob to violence. In a video posted on January 4, 2021, Charlene

Bollinger claimed that she had been working with organizers of the event, including "Ali," an apparent reference to Ali Alexander, a leader of the "Stop the Steal" movement. As the Capitol Building was being ransacked behind her, Charlene Bollinger called it "an amazing day," leading a prayer for those she called "patriots." Ty Bollinger stood at the door of the Capitol, waiting to get in. Mikki Willis, the producer of *Plandemic,* stood next to Charlene Bollinger, shouting, "Our proud patriots just pushed through a line of riot police peacefully, as peacefully as that could happen, and are now at the stairs, at the doors of the Capitol. And it is a beautiful thing to see." Charlene Bollinger screamed, "We are winning. We are at war."

Del Bigtree, another anti-vaccine activist, was also there telling the crowd, "We're being led off a cliff. I wish I could tell you that Tony Fauci cares about your safety. I wish I could tell you I believed in the CDC ... I wish I could tell you that this pandemic really is dangerous. I wish I could believe that voting machines worked ... but none of this is happening."

On June 16, 2022, anti-vaccine activist Simone Gold was sentenced to two months in prison for storming the Capitol.

Stop the steal, embrace the chaos, burn down the house, and don't get vaccinated. The anti-vaccine movement had found a new home.

WHO FUNDS THE ANTI-VACCINE MOVEMENT?

At the start of the Covid pandemic, by embracing the power and influence of social media, and armed with the political and financial backing of right-wing activists, the anti-vaccine movement was thriving, spreading misinformation at an alarming rate. By mid-September 2021, the United States was the least vaccinated member of the world's seven most populous and wealthy democracies, or "G7," which also includes the United Kingdom, Canada, France, Germany, Italy, and Japan. Although the United States accounts for only 4 percent of the world's population, it accounted for more than 20 percent of the world's Covid deaths.

In response to the growing problem, a group called the Center for Countering Digital Hate investigated those who were most responsible for misinforming the public about vaccines. They found that only 12 people or groups accounted for 70 percent of all anti-vaccine misinformation on Facebook. They also found something else. Most of the money that supported these efforts came from a rather surprising source: sales of dietary supplements, an industry that had been arguing for the same sorts of medical freedoms for decades. Following the passage of the cynically named Dietary Supplement Health and Education Act in 1994, dietary supplements became essentially an unregulated industry. In many instances, product labels claimed that supplements supported "heart health," "prostate health," or "immune health" when scientific studies had shown no such thing. This type of labeling was permitted by the 1994 law as long as the manufacturers clearly state that the product has not been evaluated by the FDA and is not intended to diagnose, treat, cure, or prevent any disease. More accurately, the act should have been called the Dietary Supplement Health and Miseducation Act.

Much as the dietary supplement industry had successfully countered the FDA, the anti-vaccine movement had successfully countered public health agencies.

WHO ARE THE LEADERS OF THE ANTI-VACCINE MOVEMENT, AND ARE COVID VACCINES AS HARMFUL AS THEY CLAIM?

On October 16, 2020, two months before Covid vaccines were available in the United States, many of the world's leading anti-vaccine activists attended a private conference to plan how to use social media to sow distrust about Covid vaccines. Seeing this as a historic moment to recruit more members to their cause, anti-vaccine activists outlined a "master narrative" centered on three themes: (1) Covid disease is not dangerous; (2) Covid vaccines are dangerous; and (3) vaccine advocates can't be trusted. The following lists some who attended that secret meeting, and who the Center for Countering Digital Hate and the *New York Times* have called the "disinformation dozen."

ROBERT F. KENNEDY, JR., the son of Senator Robert F. Kennedy and nephew of President John F. Kennedy, graduated from Harvard University in 1976, later earning his law degree from the University of Virginia.

In 2011, based on the notion that vaccines were more harmful than the diseases they prevented, Kennedy created an organization called Children's Health Defense. The year of its founding, Children's Health Defense received $13,000 in donations. One year later, in 2012, $6,000; in 2013, $24,000; and in 2014, $13,000. Children's Health Defense was on the verge of collapse. Then Kennedy followed the lead of Texans for Vaccine Choice, trumpeting vaccine freedoms while promoting vaccine harms. Donations to his organization exploded.

In 2018, Children's Health Defense received $1 million in donations; in 2019, $3 million; in 2020, $7 million; and in 2021, $15 million. The organization also built a movie studio, launched an internet TV channel, and opened branches in Canada, Europe, and Australia, translating articles into French, German, Italian, and Spanish. Kennedy continued to sharpen his message of the individual's right to reject Covid vaccines, which he claimed had killed more people than they had saved. At this point, Kennedy had millions of followers on Facebook, Twitter, and Instagram. His Facebook page alone received more than 4.7 million visits a month when it had received fewer than 150,000 visits the year before the pandemic. And his Twitter posts garnered more attention that those of CNN, NPR, and the CDC.

Why so popular? According to Similarweb, a digital intelligence company that analyzes web traffic, Children's Health Defense had become one of the most sought-after "alternative and natural medicine sites" in the world. Owing in part to its link with the dietary supplement industry, the anti-vaccine business was booming; Kennedy also benefited. His charity now pays him $497,000 a year.

Among his many anti-vaccine tropes, Kennedy claimed that "the flu shot is 2.4 times more deadly than Covid-19," that "Bill Gates wants to chip us for surveillance and transhumanism," that 5G technology "causes catastrophic biological damage," and that Covid vaccines are "the deadliest vaccines ever made." Kennedy also claimed that the Covid vaccines later licensed by the FDA were different than those that had been initially authorized through Emergency Use Authorization. Senator Ron Johnson (R-Wisconsin) echoed this unfounded claim on Tucker Carlson's program on Fox News, showing just how uninformed these men were about how vaccines are produced and regulated (see chapter 4).

In July 2020, to dissuade African Americans from being vaccinated, Kennedy claimed that "people with African American blood react differently to vaccines than people with Caucasian blood; they're much more sensitive." When baseball legend Hank Aaron died at 86 of natural causes, Kennedy called it part of a "wave of suspicious deaths among the elderly following administration of Covid vaccines." In 2021, Kennedy debuted a propaganda film targeting African Americans called *Medical Racism: The New Apartheid,* which claimed that Covid vaccines were "just one huge experiment on Black Americans."

To dissuade parents from vaccinating their children, Kennedy said, "It is criminal medical malpractice to give a child one of these vaccines." He then traveled to an Amish community in Lancaster County, Pennsylvania, to warn of the dangers of Covid vaccines, likely contributing to that community's low immunization rates.

Kennedy also wasn't above using the lure of his family's name to peddle his lies. In a promotional video in 2019 that featured members of the Kennedy family in a sailboat, he said, "You and your guest will join me for a day of sailing and a private tour of the legendary Kennedy Compound in Hyannis Port. The more you contribute, the greater your chance of winning." In one video posted in 2020, Kennedy offered trips to the Kennedy Compound on Cape Cod for his big donors. "There's always plenty of people and good conversation," he said. "If my mom decides to come, adventure is guaranteed."

Perhaps most offensive was Kennedy's constant comparison of vaccinations to the Holocaust. On December 12, 2021, he urged supporters at a rally to "wallpaper your community legally" with anti-vaccine stickers, one of which included a picture of Fauci with a Hitler mustache. On January 23, 2022, he said, "Even in Hitler's Germany, you could cross the Alps into Switzerland, you could hide in an attic like Anne Frank did. I visited East Germany with my father in 1962 and met people who had climbed the wall and escaped, so it was possible. Many died doing it, but it was possible." Jewish children in Nazi Germany, he observed, had more freedoms than children in 21st-century America. (He later apologized.)

But his message has resonated. In his book *The Real Anthony Fauci: Bill Gates, Big Pharma, and the Global War on Democracy and Public Health,* RFK Jr. argues that Anthony Fauci, scientists, and public health officials aren't honest with the American public because they are in the pockets of Big Pharma, dark money, and billionaires like Bill Gates. Kennedy's book includes a chapter with the phrase "Final Solution," another reference to the Holocaust. (*The Real Anthony Fauci* has sold more than 500,000 copies.)

In the end, most of Kennedy's vitriol was reserved for medical freedoms—specifically opposing vaccine mandates for entry into restaurants, bars, movie theaters, sporting events, and other public venues. A direct attack, he believed, on conservative values (which is ironic coming from a son of America's most revered Democratic family). "The minute they hand you that vaccine passport, every right that you have is transformed into a privilege contingent upon your obedience to arbitrary government dictates," he told a cheering crowd at a rally on January 23, 2022. "It will make you a slave."

Kennedy's family apparently didn't get the anti-vaccine message. In December 2021, his wife urged guests who attended a holiday party at his home to either get tested or get vaccinated before entry. Kennedy later claimed that he didn't know about his wife's vaccine requirement and that attendees weren't required to show proof of vaccination or testing.

For his dangerous provision of misinformation, Robert F. Kennedy, Jr., was kicked off Instagram, and Children's Health Defense was kicked off Facebook.

On April 19, 2023, at the Park Plaza Hotel in Boston, Massachusetts, RFK Jr. announced his candidacy for president of the United States. Following the announcement, Instagram reinstated his account.

JOE MERCOLA, a physician in Coral Gables, Florida, runs the most popular alternative health and dietary supplement website in the world: Mercola.com. In 2017, he claimed a net worth "in excess of $100 million."

Mercola distributes regular updates to 1.7 million followers on Facebook, 300,000 on Twitter, and 400,000 on YouTube. Before the pandemic, Joe Mercola had a long and rich history of promoting anti-science, at one time claiming that spring mattresses emit harmful radiation. In 2012, he said that tanning beds reduced the risk of cancer, selling beds with names like Vitality for $1,200 and D-lite for $4,000. In 2016, the Federal Trade Commission successfully brought a false advertising claim against Mercola's company, which he settled by paying $2.59 million in refunds to customers who had bought his tanning beds. (Tanning beds increase the risk of skin cancer.)

For Joe Mercola, the Covid pandemic was a gold mine, affording him yet another opportunity to mislead the American public. Early in the crisis, Mercola promoted his website "Stop Covid Cold," which offered hydrogen peroxide and a plant pigment called quercetin as treatments for Covid. He has also claimed that coronavirus vaccines are "a medical fraud" because they don't prevent infections, provide immunity, or stop the spread of disease. The Covid vaccine, argues Mercola, "alters your genetic coding, turning you into a viral protein factory that has no off switch."

Was Joe Mercola right? Do the mRNA vaccines made by Pfizer and Moderna alter your genetic code?

Although the notion that mRNA vaccines could alter DNA has become a frequently voiced concern among those who are hesitant to get a Covid vaccine, it is biologically impossible. First, mRNA vaccines don't possess a nuclear access signal, which would allow mRNA to enter the nucleus of a cell, where DNA resides; you can't alter DNA if you can't get to it. Second, mRNA vaccines don't have an enzyme (called reverse transcriptase) that would allow conversion of mRNA to DNA, which is the only way mRNA vaccines could alter DNA. Finally, mRNA vaccines don't have an enzyme (called integrase) that would allow them to integrate into DNA. The chance that mRNA vaccines could alter DNA is roughly the same as the chance that they could turn people into Spider-Man—which, at least according to the 1977 comic strip, can only occur if you're bitten by a radioactive spider. Also, far from having no "off switch," the spike protein generated by mRNA vaccines is produced for a few days and then stops.

Mercola is so wealthy that he generously funds other anti-vaccine groups, which continue to promote the notion that vaccines are harmful. During the past decade, Mercola has given $3.4 million to Barbara Loe Fisher's organization, NVIC, accounting for close to 40 percent of its funding. Mercola's support has allowed NVIC to run ads in AMC movie theaters, as well as on the CBS Jumbotron in Times Square. Mercola's largesse has also allowed NVIC to buy ads with the company that supplies in-flight videos to a major U.S. airline.

DEL BIGTREE heads an organization called Informed Consent Action Network (ICAN). A former producer on a television program called *The Doctors*, Bigtree now hosts *The HighWire*, a slick, magazine-style, anti-vaccine site that broadcasted to more than 600,000 followers before it was removed from Facebook and YouTube. Through different accounts, Bigtree still misinforms about 370,000 followers, arguing that people should intentionally expose themselves to Covid so they can develop immunity the way God had intended.

The goal of every vaccine is to induce the immunity that is a consequence of natural infection without paying the price of natural infection—which, in the case of Covid, was more than a million deaths in the United States by June 2023. Does Del Bigtree really believe that this is what God had intended? Bigtree has also suggested that Covid doesn't exist while at the same time arguing that people should try and catch it naturally.

Probably no one represents the hypocrisy of the anti-vaccine movement more than Del Bigtree, who introduces episodes of *The

HighWire saying, "I don't want corporate sponsors telling us what to investigate and what to say. Instead, you're our sponsors." Bigtree, it would appear, is not subject to corporate interests, unlike, as he suggests, doctors, health care professionals, and anyone else who promotes vaccines. But public records from Bigtree's organization show that its largest supporter is the Selz Foundation, which donated more than $2.9 million between 2016 and 2018—including a lifesaving donation of $100,000 in ICAN's first year. The Selz Foundation is directed by Bernard Selz, a multimillionaire investor in big drug companies like Flexion Therapeutics and Constellation Pharmaceuticals.

In 2016, after Andrew Wakefield had reinvented himself as a filmmaker, Del Bigtree helped to produce his movie, *Vaxxed,* which, through a series of parent testimonials, recycled Wakefield's debunked claim that the MMR vaccine causes autism. The closing credits of *Vaxxed* list the Selz Foundation as a contributor. The Selz Foundation has also donated $848,000 to Andrew Wakefield's Autism Media Channel. *Vaxxed* grossed $1.4 million and inspired a sequel; Robert F. Kennedy, Jr., was the executive producer.

In 2018, Del Bigtree inserted himself into a measles outbreak that swept through an ultra-Orthodox Jewish community in New York City. When the city responded with a series of increasingly more stringent vaccine mandates, Bigtree showed his distaste by having followers wear a yellow Star of David, as was forced upon Jews in Nazi Germany. Bigtree's yellow star replaced the word "Jude" (Jew) with "Vaccine." While several ultra-Orthodox Jewish children were fighting for their lives on ventilators in a New York City hospital, Bigtree pinned a Star of David on himself and sent out a press release to make sure that he received the widest possible coverage. Frankly, it is hard to imagine a crueler, more tasteless, more insensitive act. In 2020, ICAN had $5.5 million in revenue.

SHERRI TENPENNY is a physician and alternative health entrepreneur who offers paid boot camps on anti-vaccine activism. "My job is to teach 400 of you in the class," she said, "so each one of you go out and teach 1,000." For one training session on Zoom, titled "How Covid-19 Injections Can Make You Sick ... Even Kill You," participants paid $199 to attend. For another, which cost $165, Tenpenny had more than 2,000 attendees, which netted a likely profit of hundreds of thousands of dollars. Attendees at Tenpenny's boot camps learn that the Covid pandemic is a scam, that masks suppress the immune system, and that Covid vaccines are "a genocidal, DNA-manipulating, infertility-causing, dementia-causing machine." In March and April 2021, Tenpenny appeared on several QAnon shows, later tweeting about an impending transhumanist plot she believed had been orchestrated by Bill Gates, who was supposedly working on a project to block the sun. She also blamed the Sandy Hook massacre on vaccines. Like other anti-vaccine activists, Tenpenny regularly hawks dietary supplements. She also believes that Covid vaccines cause people to become magnetic.

CHARLENE AND TY BOLLINGER, a Tennessee couple who market books and videos about cancer, vaccines, and Covid, exemplify the synergy and coordination among anti-vaccine activists. They created a multimedia series called *The Truth About Vaccines* that includes "The Coronavirus Field Guide," featuring anti-vaccine stars such as Robert F. Kennedy, Jr., Andrew Wakefield, Barbara Loe Fisher, Del Bigtree, and Joe Mercola. The series, which costs up to $500, promotes intravenous vitamin C to cure Covid and links the pandemic to the 5G conspiracy that Bill Gates plans to inject everyone with microchips.

Both claims are without merit. First, an analysis of six studies involving more than 500 participants with Covid has shown that vitamin C doesn't reduce the length of hospital stay or need for mechanical ventilation, or lessen the incidence of death. Second, microchips, which are roughly the size of a grain of rice, are too large to fit through the bevel of a needle.

A portion of the proceeds from sales of this series is donated back to Robert F. Kennedy, Jr. The Bollingers claim to have sold tens of millions of dollars' worth of products through these marketing schemes and have more than a million followers on Facebook.

RASHID BUTTAR, who died in May 2023, was a physician who, appealing to parents' desperate desire to cure their children of autism, offered chelation therapy, which rids heavy metals from the body. Because heavy metals don't cause autism, Buttar had become a cottage industry of false hope. For his efforts, the FDA cited Buttar for making false claims about the treatment of a variety of disorders.

Like many anti-vaccine activists, Buttar claimed that Covid vaccines cause infertility. This fear was spawned by Michael Yeadon, a retired doctor who had worked for Pfizer, and Wolfgang Wodarg, another physician, who jointly filed a petition to the European Medicines Agency (EMA), which is the European equivalent of the FDA. Both physicians had previously declared that "the pandemic is effectively over," when it wasn't, and that Covid is no more dangerous than seasonal influenza, which, at the time, was untrue. (In the United States, influenza kills between 20,000 and 60,000 people every year. During the first two years of the Covid pandemic—when population immunity following either vaccination or natural infection was low— SARS-CoV-2 killed more than a million Americans.)

To support their claim that Covid vaccines cause infertility, Yeadon and Wodarg argued in their petition to the EMA that the

SARS-CoV-2 spike protein was virtually identical to a protein called syncytin-1, which resides on the surface of placental cells and is important for placental health. If this were true, then women making an immune response to the viral spike protein in Covid vaccines might also inadvertently make an immune response to their own placenta, causing infertility. Fortunately, SARS-CoV-2 spike protein and syncytin-1 are immunologically distinct; an immune response to one isn't also an immune response to the other.

If these doctors were right—given that more than a hundred million people in the United States have been infected with SARS-CoV-2, and that virtually all had made an immune response to the spike protein—then the birth rate should have plummeted. But the birth rate during the Covid pandemic stayed the same. Also, during the placebo-controlled, phase 3 trials of Pfizer's and Moderna's mRNA vaccines, 36 individuals got pregnant. If the Covid vaccines caused infertility, then most, if not all, of those pregnancies should have occurred in the placebo group, not the vaccine group. But the pregnancies were equally divided: 18 in the vaccine group and 18 in the placebo group, showing that the vaccines neither enhanced nor decreased fertility.

SAYER JI runs a popular alternative health website called GreenMedInfo.com, which is full of natural remedies and vaccine misinformation. Like Robert F. Kennedy, Jr., and Del Bigtree, Ji frequently evokes images of the Holocaust, stating that the rollout of Covid vaccines had a "resemblance to previous phases of human history marred by genocide." Ji claims that he no longer "critically accepts the basic tenets of classical germ theory." (The germ theory states that specific germs cause specific diseases. For example, SARS-CoV-2 causes Covid. Presumably, Sayer Ji doesn't believe this.) Ji recommends dietary supplements and avoidance of 5G networks. He has 500,000 Facebook followers and 15,000 YouTube subscribers.

MIKE ADAMS is the founder of *Natural News*. First registered in 2005, *Natural News* is the second largest alternative medicine website behind Mercola.com, garnering about 3.7 million visits a year. Links to Adams's "Health Ranger Store" are featured throughout his site, which sells dietary supplements and preparedness supplies. Like other successful anti-vaccine activists, Adams has ties to the conservative Right, guest hosting Michael Flynn and Sidney Powell—one of Donald Trump's lawyers during his attempts to overthrow the 2020 election—on his show.

Adams believes that mRNA vaccines are "extermination machines," that the pandemic vaccine rollout was a "left-wing suicide cult," and that people sickened by vaccines will be replaced by "obedient third world illegals," while those refusing vaccines will be "hunted for extermination."

Adams also claims that "vaccinated people are making healthy people sick" via "shedding of the vaccine," causing strokes, heart attacks, and infertility. No one took this claim further than a Florida educator named David Centner, who runs the Centner Academy, which carries the ironic tagline, "The Brain School."

In October 2021, five months after Covid vaccines had been approved for everyone over the age of 12, Centner prohibited vaccinated teachers from the classroom for at least 30 days because of his fear of vaccine "shedding"; a few months earlier, he had invited Robert F. Kennedy, Jr., to speak at his school. At the time of the prohibition, Centner wrote a letter to parents: "It is in the best interests of the children to protect them from the unknown implications of being in close proximity for the entire day with a teacher who has very recently taken the Covid-19 injection ... we feel it is prudent to take an abundance of caution and limit potential risk." A few months later, Centner also banned vaccinated children from attending school for 30 days.

Consider the logic of David Centner's concern about vaccine "shedding." The mRNA vaccines contain a small piece of genetic material that serves as a blueprint for a cell to make the SARS-CoV-2 spike protein. When the vaccine mRNA enters cells, it joins about 200,000 other pieces of mRNA that are making the proteins and enzymes necessary for life. If it were true that these proteins were "shed" from the body and transferred to someone else standing nearby, imagine what that could mean. People with insulin-dependent diabetes could just stand next to someone who was making insulin, freeing themselves from painful insulin injections. Or people with sickle cell disease could just stand next to someone making normal hemoglobin, no longer requiring frequent hospitalizations and blood transfusions.

Centner's prohibition of vaccinated teachers and students from school shows just how easily people can be seduced by magical thinking. Indeed, one math and science teacher at the Centner Academy urged students not to hug their vaccinated parents for more than five seconds to avoid the "shedding" problem.

BARBARA LOE FISHER, founder of NVIC and mother of the modern American anti-vaccine movement, has become strangely quiet, her voice drowned out by more vocal advocates like Robert F. Kennedy, Jr., Del Bigtree, Joe Mercola, and the Bollingers. In 2021, NVIC was removed from Facebook, Twitter, YouTube, and Instagram for repeated violations of community standards. By the end of that year,

PayPal no longer processed donations to Fisher's group. Although NVIC, according to the Center for Countering Digital Hate, "sits at the core of the established anti-vaccine movement," Barbara Loe Fisher's voice has largely faded into the background.

OTHERS WHO PROMOTE vaccine misinformation are also quick to support dietary supplements. For example, Alex Jones of Infowars, who built a following based on conspiracy theories, made his money marketing and selling nutritional supplements to the tune of about $20 million a year. Among many of Jones's claims was the argument that Covid vaccines destroy your immunity—a message that fit nicely into the dietary supplements he sold to "support immunity."

Like others who proffer anti-vaccine information, Tucker Carlson also supports the alternative medicine industry. In his case, he promoted cures for "declining virility." On May 6, 2021, Carlson said that "3,362 people apparently died after getting Covid-19 vaccines ... more people, according to VAERS, have died after getting the [Covid] shot ... than from all the other vaccines." (Anyone who worked or appeared on the set of Fox News in New York during the pandemic had to show proof of Covid vaccination. Carlson's show was based in New York City, but was often recorded from his home studio in Maine.)

Regarding the supposed deaths from Covid vaccines, Carlson was referring to a federal reporting system that is frequently misused by anti-vaccine activists called the Vaccine Adverse Event Reporting System (VAERS). The FDA and CDC jointly run the system. Here's how it works: Anyone who suspects that a serious side effect has occurred following a vaccine can fill out a one-page form online. Doctors, patients, parents, teachers, personal injury lawyers, conspiracy theorists, science deniers, and anti-vaccine activists can fill out the form. Everything that is reported will appear in the system's database, which is publicly available. If you report that following receipt of a vaccine your child turned into the Incredible Hulk, this will appear in the database, as Portland, Oregon, anesthesiologist Jim Laidler proved when he did just that.

So, when Tucker Carlson reported that more than 3,000 people had died following receipt of Covid vaccines, all that proved was that Covid vaccines don't make people immortal. Even if you get the vaccine, you might die of something else. Indeed, all these reported deaths were evaluated and found to have another cause. "There's very little control over what can be accessed and what can be manipulated [in VAERS]," says Melanie Smith, director of analysis at Graphika, a company that tracks vaccine misinformation online. Smith says that VAERS data are shared across a wide variety of anti-vaccine social media channels. "I would say almost every mis- and disinformation story that we cover is accompanied by some set of VAERS data."

The only way to know whether a vaccine causes a problem is to determine whether the problem occurs more frequently in those who are vaccinated than in those who aren't. VAERS doesn't provide that kind of information. But other federal programs, like the Vaccine Safety Datalink (VSD), do. The VSD program evaluates serious side effects in people who are vaccinated and compares them in real time to those in people who aren't vaccinated. Many of the claims made in VAERS disappear under closer scrutiny by the VSD.

Although the Covid pandemic emboldened many professional anti-vaccine activists, one stands above the rest. His voice deserves special attention because—not only was he a productive and well-respected researcher—he participated in the birth of mRNA vaccines. When this man said mRNA vaccines were dangerous, people listened.

CHAPTER 6

ROGUE SCIENTIST: THE REMARKABLE STORY OF ROBERT MALONE

- Who is Robert Malone?
- Are Robert Malone's fears about Covid vaccines warranted?
- Was Robert Malone the inventor of mRNA vaccines?

On January 23, 2022, one year after rioters stormed the United States Capitol, speakers at a "Defeat the Mandates" rally stood in front of the Lincoln Memorial. Robert F. Kennedy, Jr., informed the crowd that "if you take the vaccine, you have a 21 percent chance of dying over the next six months." Rizza Islam, an outspoken member of the Nation of Islam, said, "You used the Black community yet again to push poison." Del Bigtree said, "Mark my words. We will hold Tony Fauci accountable. We will hold Deborah Birx accountable. We will hold Joe Biden accountable."

The rally also included seven members of America's Frontline Doctors, the group that had promoted hydroxychloroquine on the steps of the Supreme Court less than two years earlier. But another doctor was there that day. Unlike the America's Frontline group, whose careers had been uninspiring at best, this doctor was different: By his own admission, he had invented mRNA technology, an achievement that should have put him in line for a Nobel Prize.

His name was Robert Malone.

Eloquent and soft-spoken, Malone began by quoting Harry Truman: "I just tell the truth, and they think it's hell." Then St. Augustine: "Truth is like a lion. You don't have to defend it. It will defend itself." He wistfully evoked the image of Martin Luther King, Jr., saying, "Honest words spoken from the heart can change the world." Then he talked about the mRNA technology he claimed to have invented. "Regarding the genetic vaccines," he said, "the science is settled. They're not working ... Whether they made sense for protecting our elderly and frail from the original virus is irrelevant." (Although surely not irrelevant to the elderly and frail.) "These are my truths," said Malone, evoking the preamble to the Declaration of Independence, "and I believe them to be self-evident." If you didn't know better, you would have assumed that Robert Malone was running for political office.

Malone then turned to the safety of the invention his work had enabled, explaining that "1 in 2,000 to 1 in 3,000 children will be hospitalized with damage caused by these vaccines." Disdaining vaccine mandates, Malone said, "If there is risk, there must be choice. We must decide for ourselves whether we willingly accept those risks." (Which assumes that you haven't been misinformed about those risks.) At the end of his 15-minute speech, to thunderous applause, Malone said that Covid "should never have been politicized."

"You tell 'em, doc," shouted a man in the crowd.

WHO IS ROBERT MALONE?

In 1981, Robert Malone studied computer science at Santa Barbara City College, later receiving his bachelor of science in biochemistry from the University of California, Davis, and his master of science in biology from the University of California, San Diego. In 1991, he graduated from Northwestern Medical School, followed by a postdoctoral fellowship at Harvard Medical School.

Before attending medical school, in the late 1980s, Malone and his co-authors published two important papers. The first appeared in the prestigious *Proceedings of the National Academy of Sciences*. Malone and his co-workers had taken a piece of mRNA that served as a blueprint for an enzyme called luciferase, put the mRNA into a fat droplet, then injected the combination into mouse cells in a lab dish. The mouse cells took up the mRNA and made the enzyme, causing cells to light up. If cells could create proteins from mRNA, Malone wrote on January 11, 1988, it might be possible to "treat RNA as a drug."

One year later, Malone repeated the experiment. This time, instead of inoculating mRNA into mouse cells in a dish, he injected the mRNA into the muscles of living mice, more closely mimicking the Covid vaccines that Pfizer and Moderna would develop 30 years later. The muscle cells made the desired protein. These two studies have been recognized as among the earliest steps in the development of mRNA vaccines.

Today, however, when newspaper, magazine, and television reporters describe mRNA vaccines, Robert Malone's name is rarely mentioned. Rather, reporters talk admiringly about Drew Weissman, Katalin Karikó, Barney Graham, Philip Felgner, Pieter Cullis, Kizzmekia Corbett, and Derrick Rossi, among others. "I've been written out of history," Malone told a *Nature* reporter. Given the importance of his earlier work, it is ironic that Malone would soon proclaim harms, real or imagined, caused by Covid vaccines.

ARE ROBERT MALONE'S FEARS ABOUT COVID VACCINES WARRANTED?

Is the Spike Protein Made by Covid Vaccines Toxic?

In November 2021, Robert Malone shared a video with his Twitter followers suggesting that a Covid vaccine had killed Jake West, a

17-year-old Indiana high school football player who had died suddenly. Malone tweeted the video to his 200,000 followers with three provocative words: "Safe and effective?"

In fact, the Covid vaccine had played no part in West's death. The teen had died from an undiagnosed heart condition in 2013, seven years *before* Covid vaccines were available. Malone later deleted the tweet after receiving a cease and desist letter from West's family, claiming that he hadn't realized the video had been doctored.

One month later, on December 16, 2021, soon after the CDC had recommended Covid vaccines for five- to 11-year-olds, Malone appeared on a Wisconsin morning news program. "Before you inject your child," he said, "a decision that is irreversible, I wanted to let you know the scientific facts about this genetic vaccine, which is based on the mRNA technology I created."

"There are three issues parents need to understand," he continued. "The first is that a viral gene will be injected into your children's cells. This gene forces your child's body to make toxic spike proteins. These proteins often cause permanent damage in children's critical organs, including their brain and nervous system, their heart and blood vessels, including blood clots, their reproductive system, and this vaccine can trigger fundamental changes to their immune system. The most alarming point about this is that once these damages have occurred, they are irreparable. You can't fix the lesions within their brain, you can't repair heart tissue scarring, you can't repair a genetically reset immune system, and this vaccine can cause reproductive damage that could affect future generations of your family."

Imagine a parent in Wisconsin hearing this from a scientist who claimed to have been the inventor of mRNA vaccine technology—the technology on which the Pfizer and Moderna vaccines were built. At the time of Malone's appearance, about 10,000 children between five and 11 years of age had been admitted to intensive care units with

Covid, 90 of whom had died from the disease. Although Covid is not nearly as fatal in young children as in older adults, the virus can still cause children to suffer, be hospitalized, and die. A choice not to get a Covid vaccine isn't a risk-free choice. Malone argued that vaccination, not Covid infection, was the greater risk.

The flaw in Malone's argument is that the spike protein the mRNA vaccines make *cannot* fuse to our cells. Normally, SARS-CoV-2 attaches to cells via the spike protein, then enters cells through a process called fusion. (The spike protein is also known as the fusion protein.)

Spike proteins made by cells following mRNA vaccination, however, are locked in a pre-fusion state, unable to fuse to cells. If spike proteins made by mRNA vaccines can't fuse to cells, then they can't directly harm cells of the heart, brain, or nervous system, as Malone had suggested.

Right-wing media quickly embraced Malone's anti-vaccine diatribes.

After appearing with Tucker Carlson, Glenn Beck, and Del Bigtree, Robert Malone was a guest on Steve Bannon's *War Room* podcast, claiming that Covid vaccines worsened outcomes in people later exposed to the virus. He laughed when he imagined the day that Tony Fauci would have to admit his mistake, saying, "Oh, darn, I was wrong!"

Bannon and Malone envisioned a future in which scientists, public health officials, and pharmaceutical company executives would finally be brought to justice for their crimes. "This is a catastrophe," Bannon beamed. "You're hearing it from an individual who invented the mRNA [vaccine] and has dedicated his life to vaccines! He's the *opposite* of an anti-vaxxer." (An anti-vaxxer is someone who promotes misinformation about vaccines causing people to put themselves, their families, and others at unnecessary risk. Robert Malone is an anti-vaxxer.)

Malone's conservative media tour continued with shows such as Fox News's *Hannity,* which garners more than three million viewers;

Candace with Candace Owens; *America First With Sebastian Gorka;* and *The Joe Pags Show.* But his career as an anti-vaccine activist took off when he appeared on the *Joe Rogan Experience,* a podcast with more than 11 million listeners per episode. In 2020, Joe Rogan signed a multiyear licensing agreement with Spotify worth an estimated $100 million, one of the largest licensing agreements in the podcast industry. On December 30, 2021, two weeks after his appearance on the Wisconsin morning news show, Robert Malone taped a three-hour interview with Rogan that aired the following day. Tens of millions of people have seen or listened to it. Malone and Rogan addressed several vaccine issues on the podcast, virtually none of which were supported by facts.

Did President Biden Fake His Covid Vaccination?

Malone and Rogan thought it was suspicious that when President Biden received his vaccine on national television, the nurse had failed to pull back on the syringe prior to injection.

> **Rogan:** *But I saw the shot where Joe Biden got it on TV, and they didn't aspirate them.*

> **Malone:** *I don't know what to say.*

> **Rogan:** *I'll tell you what to say—that's not the way to do it!*

Rogan, in addition to his experience as a comedian, actor, host of the television program *Fear Factor,* and Ultimate Fighting Champion color commentator is, apparently, also a skilled nurse.

In the past, nurses aspirated the syringe prior to injection to make sure that the needle hadn't inadvertently entered a blood vessel; this technique was abandoned in 2016, five years before Rogan's podcast, when it was found to be unnecessarily painful and essentially useless. But to Robert Malone and Joe Rogan, this meant that something fishy was going on—that President Biden hadn't really been vaccinated.

Malone and Rogan pressed on.

Do Vaccine Mandates Violate the Nuremberg Code?

> **Malone:** *These mandates of an experimental vaccine are explicitly illegal. They are explicitly inconsistent with the Nuremberg Code.*

Drafted in 1947, the Nuremberg Code outlines ethical principles for conducting medical research on human subjects. The code was created in response to experiments by Nazi Dr. Josef Mengele, which included amputating limbs and resecting organs of twins without anesthesia, killing children to obtain pathology specimens, putting prisoners in ice-cold water to monitor vital signs until they froze to death, and throwing prisoners into decompression chambers until fatal nitrogen bubbles appeared in their blood, then dissecting their brains.

At the time of Joe Rogan's podcast, the Pfizer and Moderna vaccines had been formally tested in more than 70,000 people, and fully recommended by the CDC. They weren't experimental. And they surely didn't violate the Nuremburg Code.

Is Myocarditis Following Receipt of mRNA Vaccines More Common and More Severe Than the CDC Claims?

> **Rogan:** *Now, one of the things that people have said in response to the vaccine injuries is that it's*

approximately 1 in 1,000 that are getting these
significant injuries like myocarditis.

One month after Joe Rogan said that the risk of severe injuries was 1 in 1,000, Robert Malone told a crowd at a Lincoln Memorial rally that the risk was 1 in 2,000 to 1 in 3,000. Rogan's 1 in 1,000 statistic came from a study out of Canada that was neither peer-reviewed nor published, and was eventually retracted when the flaw was exposed. Researchers had identified 32 cases of myocarditis in Ottawa between June and July 2021 out of 32,000 doses administered. From this, the researchers concluded that the risk of myocarditis following mRNA vaccines was 1 in 1,000. The actual number of doses administered, however, wasn't 32,000; it was 800,000. In other words, the rate of a serious adverse event like myocarditis following vaccination wasn't 1 in 1,000, as Joe Rogan had claimed, or the 1 in 2,000 or 1 in 3,000 that Robert Malone had claimed. It was 1 in 25,000. When the authors of the Canadian study realized their mistake, they withdrew the paper.

Many studies have since shown that people are far more likely to suffer severe and occasionally fatal myocarditis from Covid disease than from Covid vaccines, where myocarditis is typically short-lived and self-resolving (see chapter 4). But to Robert Malone and Joe Rogan, the Canadian study was worth trumpeting, even after it had been withdrawn and technically no longer existed.

During the Rogan interview, Malone reached a low point when he said that no studies of mRNA vaccines had shown that myocarditis following vaccination was mild and self-limited. To make his point, he referred to a study in Hong Kong in which researchers had actually concluded just the opposite; specifically, that myocarditis was "mild in most of the affected individuals, with only minimal treatment required and full recovery within a few days."

Perhaps no one was more impressed with Malone's appearance on Joe Rogan's podcast than Robert F. Kennedy, Jr., who offered nothing but praise. "In my experience," said Kennedy, "Malone's statements are measured and scrupulously sourced. I know him well enough to know that he would quickly and publicly correct any statement shown to be untrue." Since his appearance on Joe Rogan's podcast, Malone has publicly corrected none of these claims.

To protest Robert Malone's appearance on the *Joe Rogan Experience,* musicians such as Neil Young and Joni Mitchell abandoned Spotify. "I am doing this because Spotify is spreading fake information," wrote Young, "potentially causing death to those who believe [it] ... I want all my music off their platform. They can have Rogan or Young. Not both."

On January 10, 2022, two weeks after the podcast, more than 250 physicians signed a letter to Spotify titled, "A call from the global scientific and medical communities to implement a misinformation policy." In response, Daniel Ek, Spotify's CEO, said that his company does not take responsibility for what Rogan and his guests say, comparing the podcaster to "really well-paid rappers." "We don't dictate what they're putting in their songs, either," said Ek. At the time of Robert Malone's interview, the *Joe Rogan Experience* was the single most popular podcast in the world. Spotify later added a "content advisory" to Rogan's podcast, directing listeners to accurate information about Covid. But they didn't remove the podcast. Money talks: Musicians and doctors can walk.

A few days after it aired, YouTube and Twitter banned the Malone-Rogan interview. On January 3, 2021, Representative Troy E. Nehls (R-Texas) entered a full transcript of the interview into the Congressional Record, thus ensuring that future generations can be similarly misinformed.

Rogan's misinformation campaign didn't end with Robert Malone. A few days after the Malone interview, Rogan hosted a cardiologist named Peter McCullough, who claimed that, in documents obtained through the Freedom of Information Act, the CDC had "admitted" that Covid reinfections don't occur. "You can't get Covid twice," tweeted McCullough. (Which should be enormously comforting to the millions of Americans who have suffered Covid more than once.) A Reuters Fact Check team later found that the CDC had made no such admission.

WAS ROBERT MALONE
THE INVENTOR OF MRNA VACCINES?

Was Steve Bannon right when he said that Robert Malone was the inventor of mRNA vaccines? The short answer is no. Two critical inventions led to the Covid mRNA vaccines, neither of which Malone advanced. And both of which are worthy of Nobel Prize recognition.

First, the SARS-CoV-2 spike protein is inherently unstable, constantly changing shape, which makes it less effective as a vaccine. The spike protein had to be stabilized, fixed into a more rigid structure. Barney Graham, a vaccine researcher at NIH, and Jason McLellan, a structural biologist at the University of Texas at Austin, solved that problem by adding two stiff amino acids.

Second, if not properly modified, RNA sets off a massive inflammatory response that detracts from the desired immune response. In a collaboration that began in 1997, Drew Weissman, a researcher at the University of Pennsylvania, and Katalin Karikó, who worked at the German company BioNTech (which later partnered with Pfizer to make its vaccine), solved this problem. RNA is composed of four building blocks called nucleotides: adenine, guanine, cytosine, and uracil. Weissman and Karikó substituted a different nucleotide called pseudouridine into the viral mRNA (replacing uracil), eliminating the unwanted inflammatory response.

Perhaps more than anyone else, Katalin Karikó has been a target of Malone's ire. After CNN called her work "the basis of the Covid-19 vaccine" and a *New York Times* headline declared that she had "helped shield the world from coronavirus," Malone lamented, "It's all about Kati." In June 2021, Malone sent Karikó an email accusing her of misinforming reporters to inflate her own accomplishments. "This is not going to end well," he wrote. Karikó responded, "I have never claimed more than discovering a way to make RNA less inflammatory." In his email, Malone referred to himself as Karikó's "mentor" and "coach," though she says she had met him only once, in 1997.

Although his experiments with mRNA in the late 1980s were clearly valuable, Robert Malone didn't factor into either of the two critical advances necessary for the invention of Covid mRNA vaccines.

Nonetheless, on the anti-vaccine circuit, Robert Malone is a hero, hailed as the inventor of mRNA vaccines. His Twitter bio—before he was banned from Twitter—stated, "I literally invented mRNA technology when I was 28."

Like many anti-vaccine activists, Robert Malone has thrived during the Covid pandemic. His Substack newsletter, which has more than 134,000 subscribers, brings in an estimated $31,200 a month. According to Zignal, a media research firm, Malone was mentioned more than 300,000 times in print, cable, and social media in only the first few months of 2022. Like Robert F. Kennedy, Jr., Del Bigtree, Joe Mercola, and Charlene and Ty Bollinger, among others, Robert Malone is in the Covid misinformation business. And business is good.

ALTHOUGH HE HAD BEEN an accomplished researcher, Malone decided to burn down the house—to use his platform as one of the inventors of the mRNA vaccine technology to scare people away from using it. (Malone has been vaccinated.) In the end, Malone is wrong when he says that he has been "written out of history." History will likely remember him. But for all the wrong reasons.

Anti-vaccine activists and science denialists had an impact. Much of the suffering and deaths from Covid could have been prevented had people chosen to be vaccinated. But they believed the myths. As a result, hundreds of thousands of people died needlessly.

A PANDEMIC OF THE UNVACCINATED

- Who is most likely to reject getting Covid vaccines?
- Why do some people reject getting Covid vaccines?
- What is the best way to convince people to vaccinate moving forward?

I have been writing about the anti-vaccine movement for about 30 years. Following the false concern in 1998 about the MMR vaccine causing autism, I wrote a book called *Autism's False Prophets: Bad Science, Risky Medicine, and the Search for a Cure*. When a critical percentage of parents stopped vaccinating their children, causing sporadic outbreaks of pertussis and measles, I wrote a book called *Deadly Choices: How the Anti-Vaccine Movement Threatens Us All*.

In the process of writing these books, I spoke with a lot of people who refused to vaccinate themselves or their children. One of the main reasons they were hesitant was that they didn't see or fear the diseases that vaccines prevented. "Why does my child need a polio vaccine? Or a diphtheria vaccine? Or a pneumococcal vaccine? Or a chicken pox vaccine? I had chicken pox and I'm fine." Vaccines, it appeared, had become a victim of their own success.

That's why the rejection of vaccines during the Covid pandemic surprised me. Here was a disease that everyone saw. People were dying right in front of us. Businesses were decimated. Families were torn apart. The economy shut down. Once vaccines were available, almost all the hospitalizations and deaths from Covid were in people who had chosen not to be vaccinated. It was an unfathomable level of denialism. Health officials estimated that a choice to not get a Covid vaccine caused the deaths of about 330,000 Americans.

If we are to avoid suffering and death in the next pandemic virus—remembering that SARS-CoV-2 is the third pandemic virus in the last 20 years—then we need to understand why people chose not to vaccinate themselves or their families at a time when it was impossible to imagine how anyone could have made that choice.

THE MEDIA HAVE OFTEN characterized the divide between those who chose to accept or reject Covid vaccines at the height of the pandemic in simple terms: liberal versus conservative, Left versus Right, Democrat versus Republican, or urban versus rural. But it's not that simple.

WHO IS MOST LIKELY TO REJECT GETTING COVID VACCINES?

In April 2022, a nationwide survey by the Pew Research Center found that 73 percent of registered Democrats but only 55 percent of Republicans had been vaccinated. As a result, for the first time in human history, a person's political affiliation determined the likelihood of dying from an infection. The specifics were jarring:

- At the end of 2021, the CDC found that Montgomery County, Maryland, a heavily Democratic region just outside the District of Columbia, was *the most vaccinated county in America*. About 93 percent of people over 12 had been vaccinated, compared with 70 percent nationwide. As a result, Covid death rates in Montgomery County were eight times lower than the national average.

Other counties with vaccination rates significantly higher than the national average were Dane County, Wisconsin (home to Madison), Multnomah County, Oregon (home to Portland), Denver County, Colorado (home to Denver), Hennepin County, Minnesota (home to Minneapolis), and two counties in California: Alameda County (home to Oakland) and Santa Clara County (home to San Jose). All these counties were heavily Democratic, and all had Covid death rates three to eight times lower than the national average.

• At the beginning of 2022, the states with the highest death rates from Covid were Arizona, Mississippi, Alabama, Tennessee, and West Virginia—all of which (save Arizona) had supported Donald Trump for president. But the state with the sixth highest death rate, New Jersey, was controlled by Democrats, which had voted overwhelmingly for President Biden in 2020.

The reason for this disparity could be found in one county in central New Jersey: Ocean County, which voted for Donald Trump during the 2020 election by a 30-point margin. Only 58 percent of Ocean County residents were vaccinated, compared with the state's average of 80 percent. In the city of Lakewood, which includes many ultra-Orthodox Jewish residents, only 40 percent were vaccinated. Ocean County suffered 460 Covid deaths for every 100,000 residents—a death rate that outpaced not only every other county in New Jersey, but also almost every other county in the United States.

• Though many states encouraged people to be vaccinated, four (Florida, Kansas, Iowa, and Tennessee) rewarded people who weren't vaccinated. Officials in those four states extended benefits to workers who were fired or quit over their employers' vaccine requirements. Previously, only those who were laid off through no fault of their own could receive such benefits. In November 2021, the news website Axios reported that these policy changes were about "building loyalty with unvaccinated Americans ... a chance for Republicans to rally their base ahead of the midterms."

In the conservative movement's support of those who had chosen to remain unvaccinated, one of its lowest moments occurred during a Republican rally in October 2021, when Eric Trump's biggest applause line was, "Do you want to get a vaccine, or do you not? Do you want to be left alone, or do you not?" Don't worry, implored the younger Trump, when you choose not to be vaccinated, the Republican Party stands behind you. Also appearing at the rally was a homeopathic doctor named Edward Group who explained how drinking your own urine could ward off Covid; another speaker, Carrie Madej, said the vaccines contained a microscopic technology designed to put "another kind of nervous system inside you." "The real purpose of the vaccines," she claimed, "was to turn humans into cyborgs."

The media were quick to tell the stories of conservative legislators or pundits who had died from Covid:

• In August and September of 2021, three conservative radio talk show hosts, Dick Farrel, Phil Valentine, and Marc Bernier, died from Covid. Bernier, who had labeled himself "Mr. Anti-Vax," said that the Biden administration's push for vaccines was "Nazi-esque." Farrel had posted on Facebook, "Why take a vax promoted by people who lied to you all along about masks, where the virus came from, and the death toll?" Valentine had said he wasn't going to get vaccinated because, as a healthy 61-year-old, his chance of dying was "essentially zero."

• On November 30, 2021, Marcus Lamb, co-founder of the conservative Christian Daystar Television Network, died from Covid at the age of 64. Lamb's network had dedicated hours of programming to anti-vaccine groups such as America's Frontline Doctors and Robert F. Kennedy, Jr. Lamb's son, Jonathan, believed his father's death was a "spiritual attack from the enemy to take him down."

• On December 17, 2021, Washington State senator Doug Ericksen died from Covid after co-sponsoring a bill to prevent local governments and employers from mandating Covid vaccines.

• On December 25, 2021, Doug Kuzma, a podcaster who had opposed vaccines, died from Covid. Kuzma had contracted the disease while attending a "ReAwaken America" event in Dallas that featured Mike Lindell, Alex Jones, and Michael Flynn. Other attendees who were infected during the event claimed they had been poisoned with anthrax.

• On January 6, 2022, Cirsten Weldon, a leading QAnon promoter, who had said that "only idiots get vaccinated," and that Anthony Fauci "needs to be hung from a rope," died from Covid. Fellow QAnon members believed that Weldon had died because the hospital staff had denied her "lifesaving medications," such as ivermectin and hydroxychloroquine, and that other QAnon members who had died from Covid had been murdered by the deep state.

• On January 28, 2022, Robert LaMay, a Washington state trooper who had resigned in protest over Governor Jay Inslee's vaccine mandate for state employees, died from Covid. "Jay Inslee can kiss my ass," said LaMay, who had been lionized by Fox News stars Laura Ingraham and Maria Bartiromo, neither of whom mentioned his name after his death.

None of these stories, however, includes words like "tragedy" or "loss," which was unfortunate. No one deserves to die for their false beliefs, no matter how distasteful their politics or willful, in-your-face, or obnoxious their rhetoric.

Brytney Cobia, a hospitalist at Grandview Medical Center in Birmingham, Alabama, best described the conflicting feelings of many in the health care profession who have watched people suffer and die from bad decisions based on bad information.

On July 18, 2021, when only 33 percent of Alabamans had been vaccinated, Cobia posted an emotional message on her Facebook page:

> I'm admitting young healthy people to the hospital with very serious Covid infections. One of the last things they do before they're intubated is beg me for the vaccine. I hold their hand and tell them that I'm sorry, but it's too late. A few days later when I call time of death, I hug their family members and I tell them the best way to honor their loved one is to go get vaccinated and encourage everyone they know to do the same. They cry. And they tell me they didn't know. They thought it was a hoax. They thought it was political … They thought it was "just the flu"… And they wish they could go back. But they can't. So they thank me and they go get the vaccine. And I go back to my office, write their death note, and say a small prayer that this loss will save more lives.

Cobia struggled to find compassion. "You kind of go into it thinking, 'Okay, I'm not going to feel bad for this person, because they made their own choice.' But then you see them, you see them face-to-face, and it really changes your whole perspective ... And even though I may walk into the room thinking, 'Okay, this is your fault, you did this to yourself,' when I leave the room, I just see a person that's really suffering, and that is so regretful for the choice that they made." Before Cobia leaves the room, she asks a question. "And the one question that I always ask them is, did you make an appointment with your primary care doctor and ask them for their opinion on whether or not you should receive the vaccine? And so far, nobody has answered yes to that question."

And therein lies the problem. A problem that can be solved. But it won't be easy. Stories of those who chose not to be vaccinated show just how deeply committed some people are to that choice, and how hard it will be to use reason, logic, passion, and compassion to convince them next time. For example:

Some risked their reputation.

Kyrie Irving is an NBA star who played for the Brooklyn Nets. During the 2021–2022 basketball season, Barclays Center, where the Nets play their home games, required that anyone who entered the arena, including the players, be vaccinated. Irving refused. Consequently, he was not allowed to play in 41 home games. His refusal meant that he had to forfeit roughly half his salary—about $16 million—and dramatically weaken his team's chances of winning an NBA championship.

Novak Djokovic, a tennis star, was unable to defend his Australian Open title and was deported from Australia after refusing to be vaccinated, causing him to lose his number one ranking in the world and the possibility of winning $3 million during the tournament. Both Irving and Djokovic suffered hits to their reputation and bank accounts. Nonetheless, both held fast to their beliefs.

Some bet their lives.

Chad Carswell desperately needed a kidney transplant. "Without [a transplant] there's no telling how much longer I'll be here," said Carswell. But the Wake Forest Baptist Medical Center in Winston-Salem, North Carolina, where Carswell had been admitted, refused to provide a lifesaving kidney until he was vaccinated. When asked whether he would abide by hospital rules, Carswell said, "No sir ... I was born free. I will die free. I'm not changing my mind. I've had conversations with my family and everybody who is close to me, and they know where I stand. And there will not be a situation that occurs where I'll change my mind." Chad Carswell then bet his life that he would be able to find a hospital willing to provide a transplant to someone who wasn't vaccinated. Carswell won his bet, later receiving a kidney transplant at Duke University Hospital.

D. J. Ferguson is a father of three who was fighting for his life at Brigham and Women's Hospital in Boston. Ferguson needed a heart transplant and was high on the waiting list. But Ferguson, like Carswell, refused to be vaccinated. The hospital didn't budge, removing Ferguson from the list. (Of the 4,000 people currently on the heart transplant waiting list, 1,300 will die while waiting.)

Instead, Ferguson received a mechanical heart pump—called a left ventricular assist device—which could keep him alive for as long as five years. People who receive a heart transplant, on the other hand, live for an average of 15 years. Also, the mechanical device will take a much greater toll on Ferguson's quality of life than the transplant. "For the foreseeable future, he won't be able to shower, he won't be able to swim. He won't be able to have a life," said his father. Ferguson had chosen a shorter and lesser quality of life for fear that the vaccine would do more harm than good.

Some stories were comical.

On December 3, 2021, a 50-year-old Italian man used a fake arm to attempt to get a proof-of-vaccination card without getting a Covid vaccine. "I felt offended as a professional," said Filippa Bua, the nurse who was giving the shot. "The color of the arm made me suspicious and so I asked the man to uncover the rest of his left arm. It was well made but it wasn't the same color. At first, I thought I made a mistake, that it was a patient with an artificial arm." The man, who had two normal arms, was suspended from his work as a dentist.

Some stories were criminal.

On July 22, 2021, dozens of anti-vaccine activists, standing alongside the alt-right conspiracy groups QAnon and Proud Boys, protested outside Cedars-Sinai Breast Health Services in West Hollywood, Los Angeles, angry at the center's mandatory vaccine policy. One breast cancer patient was sprayed with bear mace, physically assaulted, and verbally abused.

In August 2021, health care workers in England received an urgent warning from Community Health Partnerships, which operates 300 health care centers across the country: "Anti-vaccination posters have been put in areas on vaccination sites that also contain hidden razor blades. When staff removes these [posters], they are being cut or injured." One 21-year-old health care worker, identified only as Layla, was tested for HIV for fear the blade that had sliced her hand was contaminated. South Wales police launched an investigation to find the perpetrators.

On November 23, 2021, Tammy McDonald, a registered nurse in South Carolina, was indicted on charges of selling fake vaccine certificates. Her attorney said McDonald used the cards to help family members who had "anti-vaccination beliefs." McDonald pleaded guilty to lying to federal agents and, although she could have faced up to five years in prison, the judge awarded her probation.

On December 30, 2021, a 37-year-old California man attacked health care workers at a vaccination site in California, calling them "murderers." One assistant was pinned down while the man delivered punch after punch. It took seven police officers 15 minutes to restrain the attacker, who was arrested and booked into the Orange County Jail. "First, we're heroes. And then somehow, we're not heroes anymore," said a spokesperson for the health center. "Now, we're the enemies." The attacker was charged with misdemeanor battery and resisting arrest.

On February 17, 2022, a Marine Corps reservist and a nurse were indicted on charges of plotting to distribute fake vaccine cards, including to other Marines who were trying to avoid the Pentagon's vaccine requirement. At the clinic, the nurse would destroy a vial of the vaccine, record the dose on the card, then enter the information into immunization databases, falsely indicating that the patient had been vaccinated, according to investigators. The scheme involved more than 300 fake vaccinations. If convicted, both men faced up to 10 years in prison. Both men subsequently pleaded guilty to conspiracy to defraud the U.S. Department of Health and Human Services. The reservist was also charged with and pleaded guilty to storming the Capitol during the January 6, 2021, insurrection.

On April 3, 2022, a German man was caught selling his vaccine certification cards after he had received 90 Covid-19 shots. At the time, vaccine certification was required in Germany to enter theaters, restaurants, swimming pools, and workplaces. Police confiscated several blank vaccination cards from the man and initiated criminal proceedings.

On November 29, 2022, Juli Mazi, a naturopath, was sentenced to 33 months in prison for selling more than 200 fake Covid vaccination cards. Mazi, who fired her attorneys and ended up representing herself, claimed that as a self-described "First Nation" person she was immune to legal action. Mazi also sold homeopathic pellets that she claimed offered "lifelong immunity to Covid-19" because they contained small amounts of the virus. Mazi didn't limit herself to Covid vaccination. Federal prosecutors alleged she also offered homeopathic pellets to children to replace other childhood vaccines and sold an additional 100 fake vaccination cards so children could attend school.

Some stories were about redemption.

On July 4, 2021, Erica Thompson, a 37-year-old mother of three in St. Louis, Missouri, died of Covid. Her mother, Kimberle Jones, said that her daughter "adamantly didn't believe in [the Covid] vaccine … and didn't believe [the disease] would ever happen to her." "She cried and cried and said, 'I want to live,'" recalled Jones. "Day after day I would go to the hospital … she developed a lot of infections, blood clots, her kidneys started shutting down … It was just heartbreaking to watch her body not respond to any medication. I just felt like my daughter, it wasn't even her." Jones said that the weeks her daughter spent in the hospital were "the most grueling, excruciating 50 days of my life."

After saying goodbye to her daughter, Kimberle Jones went on a mission, repeatedly telling her story so that all Americans, especially African Americans, would get the vaccine. "Had my daughter been vaccinated, I think she would still be here with us," said Jones. "Don't be selfish. Get vaccinated because it's not only showing you love yourself; [it's showing] you love your community, your neighbors, your employers, your co-workers. That's my prayer."

On July 27, 2021, Michael Freedy, a father of five died of Covid. "He was only 39," recalled his fiancée, Jessica. "You can't say, 'I'm young, and it won't affect me,' because it will. We wanted to wait just one year from the release to see what [side] effects people had." Jessica subsequently vaccinated herself and her children. "One of the last text messages he sent to me was, 'I should have gotten the damn vaccine ... because it would have stopped it from progressing so fast,'" she said. "I expected 30 more years with him." To find meaning in her loss, Jessica spent much of her time pleading with other families to get vaccinated.

In late 2021, Chris Crouch had a decision to make. His wife, Diana, who was 20 weeks pregnant, was in the intensive care unit and on a ventilator, struggling with Covid. Pregnant women are two to three times more likely to be hospitalized, to require intensive care, and to die from Covid than women of the same age who aren't pregnant. If the doctors delivered the baby now, Diana had a much better chance of living. But the baby was still four weeks away from surviving outside the womb. Which would Chris choose? If he allowed the pregnancy to continue, his wife might die. If he chose to deliver the child by caesarean section, his wife would likely live, but the child would likely die.

Neither Chris nor his wife had been vaccinated. When the vaccines were first available, Chris, who lived in Houston, became outspoken against them, arguing that vaccine mandates violated his personal freedoms—a point of view Texas governor Greg Abbott had promoted. "God gave us our immune system [so] we can fight the viruses," said Chris. Diana was worried about hurting her baby during the pregnancy.

As Chris Crouch watched his wife suffer, he asked himself the obvious question: "Was this my fault?" After vaccinating himself, he wrote to friends, family members, and strangers on Facebook, urging them to get vaccinated. "When you sit there and you see your wife on life support because of Covid, you throw out politics," he said later. "None of that matters anymore." Diana was placed on a heart-lung machine, which offered a 50 percent chance of survival. On November 10, 2021, when the baby boy was 31 weeks gestation, doctors delivered him by caesarean section. He weighed four pounds, 12 ounces.

Just before Christmas, on December 23, 2021, Diana returned home. She had been in the hospital for 139 days, 101 of them on a ventilator, 51 on a heart-lung machine. She still required an oxygen tank and had three chest tubes to keep her lungs expanded. But she was alive, and so was her baby.

WHY DO SOME PEOPLE REJECT GETTING COVID VACCINES?

Although it is easy to point to the cultural divide in the United States as the reason that, by the middle of 2023, about 30 percent of the population had chosen not to be vaccinated, another force is at work that is far more powerful. A force that was revealed in the answer to Brytney Cobia's last question when she asked her patients if they had talked to a doctor about their choice.

On April 8, 2022, Ed Yong, a staff writer for *The Atlantic,* appeared on a podcast called *On the Media* with Brooke Gladstone. When asked about people who had chosen not to be vaccinated, Yong replied, "That decision is also an issue of inequity." Yong explained that many people don't have access to high-quality information or to medical providers they trust. "They might live in a rural community with no doctor who they regularly talk to," said Yong. "They might not have a doctor because they're uninsured. I don't understand why it's OK to think that those people deserve to die. Just because people buy into false information doesn't mean we get to abandon them."

In support of Yong's statements, a research group called the Covid States Project found that whereas 71 percent of people who had been vaccinated trusted hospitals and doctors, only 39 percent of the unvaccinated did. In large part, this was because those who were unvaccinated had far less contact with doctors and hospitals—a finding that reflects the sorry state of health insurance in this country. The Kaiser Family Foundation found that the most powerful predictor of who remained unvaccinated wasn't age, politics, race, income, or location but the lack of health insurance, even though the vaccine was free for everyone. Those who lacked health insurance—and therefore were less likely to interact with health care professionals—were more vulnerable to misinformation.

Probably no group exemplified the importance of having health insurance more than those over 65, who were highly vaccinated. Elderly people are more likely to be Republican, more likely to watch Fox News, and more likely to be on the front lines of receiving misinformation about vaccines. But they are also far more likely to have health insurance—specifically, Medicare. And far more likely to encounter doctors and other health professionals.

Although older people were more likely to be exposed to misinformation, they were also more likely to be vaccinated. Misinformation wasn't destiny. In other words, the problem wasn't as much a deficit of knowledge as a deficit of trust: Not trusting doctors or nurses or other health care workers is much easier if you rarely interact with them.

WHAT IS THE BEST WAY TO CONVINCE PEOPLE TO VACCINATE MOVING FORWARD?

Ala Stanford was born in the Germantown section of Philadelphia to a teenage mother. A few years later, her father went off to college while her mother worked, leaving Ala alone to take care of her younger brother. Against all odds, Stanford later received her under-graduate degree from Penn State University, her medical degree from Penn State University College of Medicine, and her residency training in pediatric surgery from SUNY Downstate Medical Center and the University of Pittsburgh Medical Center, making her the first African American female pediatric surgeon to be trained entirely in the United States. "I knew I wanted to be a doctor from the time I was about eight years old," she said. "I never believed I couldn't do it."

Stanford spent the early days of the pandemic providing Covid tests to communities of color. "For us, it doesn't matter what type of insurance you have or don't have," said Stanford. "You're going to see the same people, you're going to get the same level of care, and that's what we plan to deliver for everyone who comes into the door." Although Black and Latinx residents were suffering Covid dispro-portionately, Stanford noted that most of the testing sites were in affluent white neighborhoods. "There was no testing in the commu-nities where people were dying the most. So, we created it," she said. With a rented van and personal protective equipment taken from her office, Stanford traveled to church parking lots and started swabbing noses. In April 2020, her mobile operation turned into the nonprofit group Black Doctors Covid-19 Consortium (BDCC), which grew to include 70 employees and more than 200 volunteers, all funded by Stanford. "This was a working-class community," she recalled. "They were keeping the city and the country running. But wherever Black people were, one thing that was tough to come by was testing."

Stanford's efforts were immediately successful. "The first day we did a dozen tests. The second time we went out, we did about 150 tests. And the third time there were 500 people lined up before we started." By August 2020, Stanford and her team were testing more than 1,000 people a day.

In January 2021, when Covid vaccines became available, Stanford and the BDCC started vaccinating, sometimes hundreds of people a day. The group also ran a 24-hour Vax-A-Thon, during which more than 4,000 people were vaccinated. By May 2021, the BDCC had vaccinated more than 46,000 Philadelphians, drawing praise from U.S. Surgeon General Vivek Murthy, who said, "[Stanford] is a perfect example of how a community member can stand up and lead during a time of crisis."

Stanford was successful because she sat in people's living rooms and offered a doctor who looked like them and was willing to spend time listening to their fears and concerns. "It's my job to educate and allow you to make an informed decision about your health," said Stanford. "So, I listen to what the reason is why they're not getting vaccinated. Sometimes it's lack of education; sometimes it's fear; sometimes they can't even tell you why. Sometimes the questions they have, there are no answers for. So, I just state the facts, and I'm honest with them. But you're more likely statistically to die if you're African American and you contract coronavirus. That is a fact. Regardless of how much money you make or not, regardless of comorbid conditions or not.

"I tell them, 'You have to weigh the risks and benefits,' and I'm available to listen and answer. It's not a one-time conversation for some people. Some people need to come back and watch a couple of people get it. And then they're like, 'OK, Doc. I'm ready.' Our mission has always been about getting Black and Brown communities the access and care they deserve."

By August 2021, Stanford and the BDCC had administered more than 50,000 vaccinations and 25,000 tests. As a result of her efforts, *Forbes* magazine recognized her as a woman over 50 who was changing the world, *Fortune* magazine named her one of the country's 50 Greatest Leaders, and CNN dubbed her a Top 10 Hero.

If we are to increase vaccine rates during the next pandemic, we need to find people like Ala Stanford who are willing to go into communities where vaccine rates are low—such as Native American, Amish, ultra-Orthodox Jewish, rural, and Black and Brown communities, among others—and sit down in living rooms and answer questions and concerns. We need to find a thousand more Ala Stanfords who, instead of vaccinating 50,000 people, vaccinate 50 million.

The good news? It's possible. It will no doubt take time and patience, but it's possible. The problem isn't going to be solved at the federal or state level. It will only be solved at the local level.

A FEW YEARS AGO, I spoke at a public health symposium in Connecticut. I described a series of studies showing that the MMR vaccine didn't cause autism. When I finished, a woman in the audience came up to the podium and screamed loudly at me for about 10 minutes, telling me that I didn't know what I was talking about. On the ride back to the train station, one of the organizers said to me, "You know you've gotten to the center of things when you meet the very best people and the very worst people."

Such has been the case with the Covid pandemic. It is hard to imagine a more striking example than the relative efforts of Dr. Ala Stanford and Robert F. Kennedy, Jr.

Stanford, the child of a 14-year-old mother in Philadelphia, rose from poverty to become a pediatric surgeon. When the pandemic hit, she set aside her practice and funded a coalition that vaccinated and tested tens of thousands of people in marginalized Black and Brown communities in North Philadelphia. No doubt saving lives.

Robert F. Kennedy, Jr., is the son of one of the most revered Democratic senators in American history. The product of a wealthy, powerful family, he chose to proffer false information about vaccines, especially to communities of color. His film, *Medical Racism: The New Apartheid,* is specifically targeted to Black communities to lower Covid vaccination rates. No doubt costing lives.

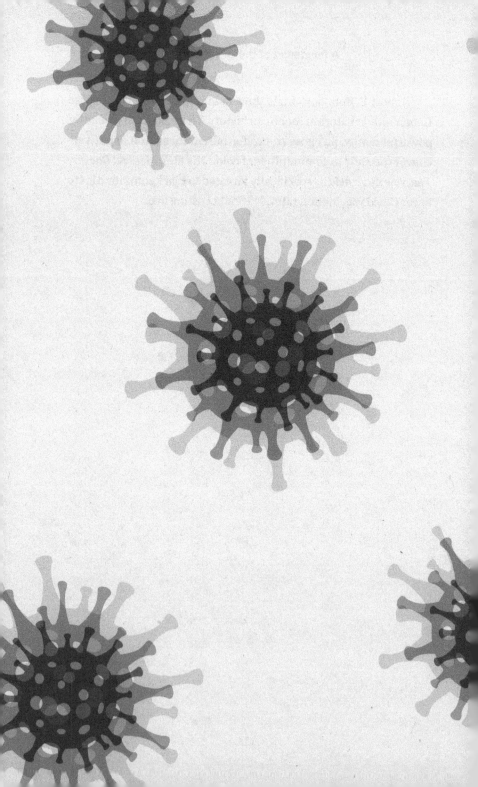

PART II

········

WHERE
WE ARE

CHAPTER 8

BOOSTER CONFUSION: WHO IS PROTECTED?

• How effective are Covid vaccines?

• What was the first major communications error regarding Covid vaccines?

• What was the second major communications error regarding Covid vaccines?

• What single event led to the birth of Covid vaccine booster doses for all?

• What was the third major communications error regarding Covid vaccines?

• Does frequent booster dosing with Covid vaccines have a downside?

In 2020, after the approval of hydroxychloroquine for treatment of Covid, many Americans lost faith in the FDA and the White House. This erosion in faith didn't end with the Trump administration. Because of a series of communication errors in 2021 and 2022, many also started to lose faith in the CDC and the Biden administration. Consequently, by the beginning of 2023, Americans were confused about how many doses of Covid vaccine were necessary for protection. Who was benefiting from all these boosters?

HOW EFFECTIVE ARE COVID VACCINES?

Some viral vaccines are so good that they can prevent even mild illness for decades and eliminate the virus from the face of the planet.

Others are good at protecting against serious disease, but not as good at protecting against mild disease or spread. The difference has nothing to do with the intelligence of the scientists who invented the vaccines or the competence of the companies that make them. Rather, the effectiveness of vaccines is largely determined by one thing: the incubation period of the disease, which is the time between exposure to a virus and the onset of symptoms.

If incubation periods are long (meaning a couple of weeks, as for smallpox, measles, and polio), then the disease can be eliminated. If incubation periods are short (meaning only a few days, such as for SARS-CoV-2, influenza, respiratory syncytial virus, or other common cold viruses), then the virus is likely to circulate for centuries, causing mild illness in most and severe disease in some.

Why do incubation periods determine the effectiveness of a vaccine?

First, we need to understand which parts of the immune system are required to prevent mild illness and which are required to prevent severe illness; they aren't the same. But before we do that, we need to define what we mean by mild and severe disease.

The CDC describes severe Covid as symptoms requiring admission to a hospital or intensive care unit, and mild illness as anything less than that. Because severe Covid often affects the lungs, causing pneumonia, people with severe illness almost always require supplemental oxygen. People with mild illness—even if they are miserable, cough, have days of fever, and believe they are suffering the worst infection of their lives—don't require supplemental oxygen because the virus hasn't infected their lungs. Therefore, at least according to the CDC, they aren't severely ill.

The key determinant for protection against mild illness is the level of virus-specific antibodies present in the bloodstream at the time of exposure to the virus. The good news is that both natural infection and vaccination readily induce these antibodies. The bad news is that they don't last very long—usually three to six months—before they fade away. Therefore, for diseases with short incubation periods, protection against mild illness is always short-lived. Always.

SARS-CoV-2 vaccines are a perfect example of what you can expect from antibodies. When researchers from Pfizer and Moderna presented the results of their mRNA vaccine trials in December 2020, they showed that two doses induced 95 percent protection against mild, moderate, and severe disease, which was amazing. Why was protection against mild illness so high? The answer is that these studies were performed over a three-month period; most of the participants had just received their second dose. For that reason, everyone still had high levels of antibodies in their bloodstream and, therefore, were protected against mild disease.

But protection against mild illness couldn't last.

By the middle of 2021, about six months after people had received their second dose of vaccine—when antibodies had begun to decline—protection against mild illness had also declined from 95 percent to 50 percent.

Protection against severe illness, on the other hand, had remained high. That's because protection against severe illness isn't dependent on antibodies present at the time of exposure; it's dependent on immunological memory cells, like memory B cells, which can be stimulated to make antibodies. The good news about memory B cells is that they are long-lived, often for decades. The bad news is that these memory cells need time after exposure to the virus to become activated and make antibodies.

For diseases with short incubation periods, like Covid, symptoms begin *before* these memory B cells have time to make antibodies. Therefore, people suffer mild illness. Whereas mild Covid infections occur only a few days after exposure, developing severe disease takes much longer—about a couple of weeks. That's plenty of time for these memory B cells to become activated and make antibodies. This is why protection against mild disease is short-lived and protection against severe disease is long-lived for diseases with short incubation periods.

For diseases with long incubation periods, on the other hand, these memory B cells have more than enough time to make antibodies to prevent even mild illness. This is why it's possible to virtually eliminate diseases like smallpox, polio, and measles.

But another part of the immune system that most people don't know about is also important: T cells. These cells are divided into two groups: helper T cells, which, as their name suggests, help B cells make antibodies, and cytotoxic T cells, which kill virus-infected cells ("cytotoxic" means toxic to cells).

T cells are different than B cells. Unlike antibodies, T cells recognize parts of SARS-CoV-2 that are similar among all the different variants. Whereas new viral variants (like Omicron) escaped recognition by antibodies, they didn't escape recognition by T cells. That's because the immunologically distinct regions (epitopes) recognized by T cells remained relatively stable (conserved) across variants, from Alpha to Delta to Omicron. Memory T cells, like memory B cells, are also long-lived and provide long-term protection against serious disease.

Although antibodies induced by the vaccines made in 2020 weren't very good at recognizing the Omicron variants, T cells continued to recognize the new variants and continued to protect against severe disease. This explains why, when Omicron first entered the United States in late 2021, the number of cases of mild illness in people who had been vaccinated or previously infected was proportionally far greater than the number of hospitalizations and deaths. For otherwise healthy, young people, T cells continued to protect against severe disease; these cells weren't fooled by the Omicron variants. Only the antibodies were fooled. (Dan Barouch, an immunologist at Harvard Medical School, called T cells "the unsung hero of this pandemic.")

WHAT WAS THE FIRST MAJOR COMMUNICATIONS ERROR REGARDING COVID VACCINES?

On July 4, 2021, thousands of men gathered in Provincetown, Massachusetts, to celebrate Independence Day. Most had received two doses of a Covid vaccine. Nonetheless, 346 men who had been fully vaccinated developed Covid; four of them (1.2 percent) were hospitalized. The 342 men who weren't hospitalized developed either asymptomatic or mild infections. The Covid vaccines were working well, keeping these men out of the hospital.

This was an opportunity for the CDC to celebrate how well these vaccines were working.

Unfortunately, the CDC's report of the Provincetown outbreak gave birth to a term that misled the public. The description of the outbreak, which appeared in a CDC publication called *Morbidity and Mortality Weekly Report,* was titled, *Outbreak of SARS-CoV-2 Infections, Including Covid-19 Vaccine Breakthrough Infections, Associated with Large Public Gatherings—Barnstable County, Massachusetts, July 2021.* This was the first time that mild or asymptomatic infections had been described as "breakthroughs."

The word "breakthrough" implies failure. But Covid vaccines hadn't failed. Quite the opposite: They had succeeded in keeping almost all these men out of the hospital. In its use of the word "breakthrough," the CDC had inadvertently set a bar for Covid vaccines that was impossible to reach. From this point forward, public health officials and the media often talked about "waning immunity" without differentiating between waning protection against mild illness and waning protection against severe disease. "I got the vaccine," lamented some. "And now I have Covid. The CDC lied to me."

A few months after the CDC reported the outbreak in Province-town, Massachusetts, Supreme Court Justice Brett Kavanaugh tested positive for Covid during a routine screening. He had no symptoms. The immediacy, breathlessness, and alarm with which the media covered his story, often using the CDC term "breakthrough," caused some casual observers to conclude that Brett Kavanaugh must have been fighting for his life. One politician got it right: Lindsey Graham, a Republican senator from South Carolina—who had received two doses of vaccine—suffered a short-lived Covid infection with mild sinusitis. "This would have been much worse if I hadn't been vacci-nated," he said. Right. Exactly right.

WHAT WAS THE SECOND MAJOR COMMUNICATIONS ERROR REGARDING COVID VACCINES?

Two weeks after the Provincetown outbreak, the Biden administra-tion made its second major communications error.

On August 18, 2021, President Biden stood in front of the Amer-ican public and declared that beginning the week of September 20, 2021, booster doses would be available for everyone over 12 years of age. Biden had just told Americans that the two doses of Covid vaccine they had received weren't enough when all the evidence at the time had shown that two doses had continued to protect against severe disease for all age groups.

Why, then, did the Biden administration offer a booster dose for everyone? And why did the administration make this announcement to the American public before consulting with FDA and CDC advisory committees? When administration officials were asked to explain this sudden change in recommendations, they said, "Wait until you see the data coming out of Israel. Then you'll understand."

On September 17, 2021, one month after President Biden made his announcement and a few days before his "boosters for all" plan was set to launch, the FDA's vaccine advisory committee was asked to vote on this new directive. Before we voted, however, two Israeli researchers presented data that were supposed to provide a clear reason for why the Biden administration had said that all adults needed a booster dose.

Here's what our FDA vaccine advisory committee learned. During the previous few months, Israeli health officials had offered a booster dose of Pfizer's mRNA vaccine to anyone who wanted it. Some people in Israel took the booster dose; some didn't. The study involved thousands of Israelis, 75 percent of whom were more than 70 years old. Researchers found that 7.5 percent of those between 70 and 79 years of age who didn't get a booster dose developed serious Covid disease, whereas only 1.3 percent of those who did get the booster dose became seriously ill.

This was a striking difference. But the data was flawed. This wasn't a controlled study. Israeli researchers had assumed that those who chose the booster dose were the same as those who didn't. But it is likely that those who chose to be boosted were more attentive to their general health, more likely to wear masks and social distance, and less likely to engage in activities that put them at higher risk of Covid. Despite these obvious limitations, our committee voted to authorize a booster dose of Covid vaccine for all Americans over 65. A week later, the CDC agreed. The first booster dose was born. But only for the elderly.

Why did President Biden want to boost everyone over 12? Why didn't he just offer a booster dose for elderly Americans, who were clearly at highest risk? What were those Israeli data that were supposed to be so convincing?

At the same September 17, 2021, meeting of the FDA's vaccine advisory committee, Israeli public health officials explained that they had offered a booster dose to everyone over 16, not just the elderly. Consequently, the incidence of Covid had started to decline in Israel. But the incidence of Covid had also started to decline in the United States, which hadn't offered a booster dose to all adults. So, the more likely explanation for the decline of cases in Israel was the random fluctuations of Covid in the face of evolving variants, changing patterns of behavior among citizens, and seasonal variations, not a booster dose. For that reason, our committee voted unanimously to reject the Biden administration's plan to boost everyone over 12, as did the CDC advisory committee one week later. When President Biden took office, he vowed to "follow the science." But his administration's push in August 2021 for a booster dose for everyone over 12 hadn't made good on that promise.

By using the term "breakthrough" to describe a mild or asymptomatic illness and by sending the message that two doses of Covid mRNA vaccines weren't enough, public health officials and the Biden administration had inadvertently damned a vaccine that was working remarkably well. The terms that were subsequently used to describe the vaccine were equally confusing. Those over 65 who had received two doses of the vaccine were considered "fully vaccinated," and those over 65 who had received a booster dose were considered "up to date." This confusion would only worsen as more booster doses were recommended.

At the end of December 2021, one year after Covid vaccines had been approved in the United States, the CDC published a study of 8,000 immunocompetent adults who either had or hadn't been vaccinated with two doses of mRNA vaccines. The average age of participants in the study was 60, and more than 80 percent had at least one health problem that put them at risk of severe Covid. In this study,

CDC researchers found that protection against severe illness following two doses of vaccine remained excellent, ranging between high 80 percent to low 90 percent. Similarly, immunologists showed that the levels of memory B cells and memory T cells in the bloodstream after two doses had remained high. In other words, the immunological results were consistent with the epidemiological results showing continued protection. These studies further undermined the claim the Biden administration made several months earlier that all Americans over 12 years of age need a booster dose.

At the start of the pandemic, researchers and public health officials weren't sure how well or for how long these new mRNA vaccines would work. But one year after they had become available, protection against severe illness afforded by two doses remained high. Then, at the end of December 2021, something happened that dramatically changed the way we looked at this pandemic. Consequently, by the beginning of 2022, most Americans would have little understanding of how many doses of vaccine were necessary to protect against Covid.

WHAT SINGLE EVENT LED TO THE BIRTH OF COVID VACCINE BOOSTER DOSES FOR ALL?

In December 2021, a variant called Omicron (BA.1) entered the United States. To understand how this variant altered recommendations for booster dosing, we need to go back to the beginning.

In December 2019, in Wuhan, China, a bat coronavirus entered the human population. By January 2020, the strain had been isolated, and its genome sequenced. It was called the Wuhan-1 or ancestral strain. All vaccines, including those made by Pfizer, Moderna, Johnson & Johnson, and Novavax, were designed to protect against this strain of virus. The Wuhan-1 strain, however, wasn't the virus that left

China. The strain that would soon travel the world—the very first variant—had one critical change that stabilized SARS-CoV-2 and made it 10 times more contagious. This new variant didn't have a Greek letter designation. It was called the D614G variant.

To understand why the D614G variant was designated this way, we need to take a trip back to high school chemistry class. The SARS-CoV-2 spike protein, like all proteins, is composed of a string of amino acids. (Twenty different amino acids, with names like leucine, proline, valine, glycine, and aspartic acid, make up all proteins. Each amino acid is assigned a single letter designation. For example, aspartic acid is assigned the letter "D," and glycine the letter "G.")

The SARS-CoV-2 spike protein is 1,273 amino acids long. One change in one amino acid at position 614 (from aspartic acid [D] to glycine [G]) in the middle of the spike protein accounted for this dramatic change in contagiousness. Just one amino acid was all it took to stabilize the virus. This single amino acid change allowed SARS-CoV-2 to sweep across Asia, Europe, and the United States, killing hundreds of thousands of people.

In the United States, the D614G variant was soon replaced by the Alpha variant, then the Delta variant because each was more contagious. Other highly contagious variants, with Greek letter designations such as Gamma, Epsilon, Zeta, Eta, Theta, Iota, Kappa, Lambda, and Mu, also circulated throughout the world. (The Greek alphabet has only 24 letters, one of the smallest alphabets in modern use. The last letter in the Greek alphabet is omega. An Omega variant doesn't yet exist, but it's probably only a matter of time.)

When the Omicron (BA.1) variant reared its head, it didn't have just a handful of changes; it had 37 critical changes in the spike protein alone, far more than any previous variant. And this Omicron variant wasn't just more contagious; it was more immune evasive. This meant that even if you had been recently vaccinated or naturally infected and had a high level of antibodies in your bloodstream, you still might get a mild Covid illness because those antibodies didn't recognize the Omicron variant particularly well.

The good news was that the regions on the spike protein recognized by T cells on Omicron hadn't changed much, so people who had been previously vaccinated or naturally infected were still protected against severe disease caused by Omicron. But Omicron caused a dramatic increase of cases in people who had considered themselves to be protected against all symptomatic illness. The Omicron variants were also resistant to monoclonal antibodies. The immune evasiveness of Omicron scared public health officials.

During the next few months, in early 2022, Omicron (BA.1) continued to evolve, creating a series of subvariants with names like BA.2, BA.3, BA.4, and BA.5, each of which was more contagious and more immune evasive than the last. For example, people who had been infected with the original Omicron (BA.1) variant were still at risk of infection with BA.4 and BA.5. Again, if these people had been previously vaccinated or infected, infections were usually mild, not severe. This was also true for later Omicron subvariants with an alphabet soup of names like BQ.1, BQ.1.1, BF.7, BA.4.6, BA.2.75.2, XBB.1, XBB.1.5, and XBB.1.16.

To determine whether people benefited from a booster dose of a Covid vaccine during the Omicron wave, scientists and public health officials performed a series of studies. They found that three doses were better than two at preventing hospitalizations. Later, and to a lesser extent, they found that four doses were better than three at preventing hospitalizations. But who was benefiting from these additional doses? Was everyone benefiting or just certain groups? Who, exactly, was being kept out of the hospital?

As it turned out, not everyone equally benefited from the third and fourth doses. For the most part, booster doses were protecting the elderly (those over 75); people with severe immune deficiencies; and people who had health problems that put them at high risk of serious Covid, like severe lung, heart, or kidney disease, where even a mild infection could land them in the hospital. Pregnant women also benefited. While the CDC was studying the value of booster dosing, researchers in the United Kingdom studied more than 30 million people who either had or hadn't received a booster dose. Like the CDC researchers, the U.K. researchers found that those being kept out of the hospital were more than 80 years old, had five or more health problems, or were immune deficient.

On September 1, 2022, the CDC recommended that everyone more than 12 years of age receive a booster dose, even though the studies at the time (including those the CDC performed) had shown that booster dosing prevented severe disease in only certain high-risk groups.

At this point in the pandemic, however, booster doses had changed; they no longer contained only the original, ancestral (Wuhan-1) strain. Now, they were two vaccines in one—a so-called bivalent vaccine—containing both the ancestral strain, which had been the sole component in vaccines since December 2020, as well as a vaccine designed to protect against two almost identical Omicron variants that were circulating (BA.4 and BA.5). On October 12, 2022, the CDC extended the recommendation for a bivalent vaccine booster to include everyone over five years of age, and later to all children down to six months of age.

On the surface, the strategy of including a vaccine directed against the current circulating strains made sense. Why continue to boost with the Wuhan-1 ancestral strain when Wuhan-1 had disappeared and different strains were circulating? Now, with higher levels of antibodies against BA.4/BA.5 following vaccination, people would presumably not only be protected against severe disease but also better protected against mild disease caused by these newer Omicron variants, at least for a little while. Unfortunately, it didn't work out that way. This led to the third major communications error regarding Covid vaccines.

WHAT WAS THE THIRD MAJOR COMMUNICATIONS ERROR REGARDING COVID VACCINES?

In mid-October 2022, when the CDC recommended a bivalent booster dose for everyone over five years of age, no human data were available to prove that boosting with the bivalent vaccine (which contained both the BA.4/BA.5 strain and the Wuhan-1 strain) was better than boosting with the monovalent vaccine (which contained only Wuhan-1). One week after the recommendation was issued, the first human data appeared. Researchers at Columbia and Harvard published studies comparing the relative ability of a bivalent vaccine and a monovalent vaccine to make antibodies that neutralized BA.4/BA.5. What they found was surprising. No difference.

The Biden administration, FDA, and CDC assumed the bivalent vaccine would be much better at inducing antibodies against these newer variants. It made sense that a vaccine containing BA.4/BA.5 would induce higher quantities of antibodies against BA.4/BA.5 than a vaccine that only contained the ancestral strain.

But it didn't work out that way.

Therefore, it was unlikely that the bivalent vaccine would perform better than the monovalent vaccine. Indeed, two previous studies—one in the United States and the other in the United Kingdom—had shown that a bivalent vaccine containing BA.1 wasn't better at preventing Covid than the monovalent vaccine during a BA.1 outbreak. In March 2023, a study performed in France in people over 60 found that the BA.4/BA.5-containing bivalent vaccine increased protection against symptomatic infection by only 8 percent. Nonetheless, the Biden administration and public health officials at the FDA and CDC held fast to the claim that the bivalent vaccine was better. Much better. Dramatically better. Even though it wasn't.

Most Americans chose not to get the bivalent vaccine booster. By April 2023, seven months after the CDC had recommended the bivalent vaccine for everyone over six months of age, only 17 percent of the population for whom it was recommended chose to get it. Again, distrust of the FDA, CDC, and White House—mixed with a healthy dose of booster fatigue—had impacted vaccine uptake.

The bivalent BA.4/BA.5 vaccine launched in mid-2022 was a lost opportunity. Although no clear evidence showed it was better than the monovalent vaccine at preventing Covid, it wasn't worse. Studies showed that the bivalent vaccine prevented hospitalizations in the elderly and other high-risk groups. Whether you chose the monovalent vaccine or the bivalent vaccine, the boosters boosted.

At this point, the administration should have backed away from the claim that the bivalent vaccine was significantly better than the monovalent vaccine and simply promoted the booster dose for those at highest risk. No other country recommended booster dosing for everyone, only for those at highest risk. This episode further eroded the trust of the American public. Worse, some scientists, clinicians, and local health officials also started to lose a little faith in those making recommendations. I was one of them.

On February 9, 2023, I published an article in the *New England Journal of Medicine* titled, "Bivalent Covid-19 Vaccines—A Cautionary Tale." The final paragraph stated, "Booster dosing is probably best reserved for the people most likely to need protection against severe disease … In the meantime, I believe we should stop trying to prevent all symptomatic infections in healthy, young people." Many in the public health community applauded this stance. Some, however, were angry about my publication. And angrier still that I had appeared on national television programs countering the CDC recommendation to boost everyone. They argued that my dissent only emboldened anti-vaccine activists. It made us look like we didn't know what we were doing. That we were divided.

I see this differently. I think we should always be able to question the science behind public health recommendations. And this questioning should occur in the open, so that the public and the press can best understand the strengths and weaknesses behind specific recommendations. Every recommendation has strengths and weaknesses. If we fear public debate, then anti-vaccine activists really have won.

DOES FREQUENT BOOSTER DOSING WITH COVID VACCINES HAVE A DOWNSIDE?

By the beginning of 2023, the United States had entered a phase that some people called "boostermania." (Evidence of the public's concern about booster dosing could be found in a humorous meme titled "Pfizer Loyalty Card," a fake punch card showing that recipients of an eighth booster dose of Pfizer's vaccine could receive a free pizza.) The concern was that we had drifted away from the original goal of preventing severe disease in those at highest risk and drifted toward trying to prevent mild illness in everyone—which was, for all practical purposes, impossible. Those who supported frequent boosting argued it couldn't hurt: the "chicken soup" argument.

Like all medical products, however, anything that has a benefit can have a risk. And although those risks are acceptable when the benefits are clear, they aren't acceptable when the benefits are less clear. For example:

Law of Diminishing Returns

Researchers in Israel found that a fourth booster dose increased protection against mild Covid illness by about 50 percent. Unfortunately, three to six months later, enhanced protection against mild illness had disappeared. This was true for both children and adults. Boosting every few months to maintain protection against a short-lived, mild illness is not a viable public health strategy. Preventing severe disease is the goal of the vaccine, which appears to be relatively long-lasting in healthy young people following either three doses of mRNA vaccine or two doses plus a natural infection. (The rationale for this recommendation can be found in chapter 13, which describes the relative value of natural infection versus immunization in providing long-term protection against Covid.)

Serious Adverse Events

The mRNA vaccines are a rare cause of myocarditis (inflammation of the heart muscle) in young people, especially boys and men (see chapter 4). Though myocarditis is often short-lived, transient, and self-resolving, this might not always be the case.

Imprinting

In 1960, an influenza vaccine researcher named Thomas Francis coined the term "original antigenic sin," which today is called "imprinting." Francis observed that the first strain of influenza virus to which children were exposed determined how they would respond to influenza infections or influenza vaccination for the rest of their lives. They would, it seemed, always respond as if they were being exposed to that first strain, not recognizing the subtle differences in influenza as the virus continued to evolve.

This is already happening with Covid vaccines. One explanation for why the bivalent vaccine booster containing BA.4/BA.5 didn't induce significantly higher levels of antibodies against BA.4/BA.5 than the monovalent vaccine containing only the ancestral strain was that people had imprinted to the original ancestral strain. When the bivalent vaccine contained both the original strain and BA.4/BA.5, people responded much better to the original strain in the bivalent vaccine, because they had already been primed to do so. They had locked in to responding to the regions of BA.4/BA.5 that were identical to the ancestral strain and failed to recognize the regions on BA.4/BA.5 that were different. This could possibly be overcome by eliminating the ancestral strain from the vaccine and giving higher quantities of mRNA consistent with the circulating strains.

Another example of imprinting can be found in the first human papillomavirus (HPV) vaccine, which was designed to prevent head, neck, anal, and genital cancers. Called HPV4, the vaccine contained four different HPV strains. It was later replaced by HPV9, which contained five additional types. Adolescents who only received HPV9 developed excellent immune responses to all nine types. However, adolescents who received HPV4, then HPV9, responded better to the four types in HPV4 than the additional five types in HPV9. They had imprinted on the first four HPV types. They had locked in to the four serotypes in HPV4.

Money Better Spent

By the beginning of 2023, the federal government was continuing to pay for Covid vaccines. For example, the government spent hundreds of millions of dollars on a BA.4/BA.5-containing bivalent booster vaccine offered in the fall of 2022 that was of no apparent benefit over the monovalent vaccine. Wouldn't this money have been better spent on funding strategies to increase vaccine acceptance for those who were unvaccinated? Or by providing vaccines to developing countries?

CHAPTER 9
....

TREATING COVID

• What are the stages of Covid?
• Which Covid treatments work best at each stage?
• Which Covid treatments should be avoided?
• What Covid treatments are likely to be available in the future?

WHAT ARE THE STAGES OF COVID?

Covid occurs in two stages. In the first stage, the virus is dominant. In the second stage, the immune system takes over. Each stage requires a different treatment.

SARS-CoV-2 enters the body in tiny droplets spread from the nose and mouth by someone who is infected. The virus then attaches to and enters cells that line the nose, throat, windpipe, breathing tubes (bronchi), and, in the most severe cases, lungs.

After the virus enters cells, it begins to reproduce itself. Whereas one virus particle might enter a cell, about 100 leave the cell before killing it. Hundreds of viruses become thousands of viruses that become millions of viruses. (At this point, most people don't have any symptoms.) After a few days, the body's immune system begins to respond. B cells make antibodies and helper T cells assist. Cytotoxic T cells kill virus-infected cells. The war is on.

Although it might seem surprising, symptoms don't become obvious until the immune system kicks in, because the immune system, and not the virus alone, causes them. Once the immune system begins to fight back, viral reproduction becomes a much smaller part of the disease process, as is true for many infectious diseases. People are most contagious a day or two *before* symptoms begin, when virus reproduction is at its peak.

Because viral reproduction dominates the first stage, the best way to treat people in the first few days of illness is to give therapies directed against the virus, such as antiviral drugs (which decrease viral reproduction), monoclonal antibodies (which prevent the virus from attaching to cells), and convalescent plasma (which does the same thing that monoclonal antibodies do). During the second stage, however, when patients are severely ill and the generation of new virus particles is no longer as important, medicines directed at the virus don't work. At that point, only drugs that dampen the immune system, like steroids, are effective.

The stories of two presidents with Covid show just how much we learned during the first two years of the pandemic.

On October 1, 2020, President Donald Trump, 74 years old and overweight, tested positive for Covid. The following day, he was flown to Walter Reed National Military Medical Center for treatment. Trump's fever was high, he was short of breath, and the level of oxygen in his bloodstream (red blood cells carry oxygen from the lungs to the rest of the body) was dangerously low—all signs of severe pneumonia. Before traveling to the hospital, doctors administered a monoclonal antibody preparation called Regeneron intravenously, beginning a five-day course. (The FDA authorized Regeneron about a month later.)

When Trump arrived at Walter Reed, his chest x-ray confirmed that he was suffering from pneumonia. The severe inflammation in his lungs made it difficult for him to breathe and prevented the transfer of oxygen from his lungs to his bloodstream. Doctors administered an antiviral medicine called remdesivir. Remdesivir prevented SARS-CoV-2 from reproducing itself. (The FDA licensed remdesivir later that month.) Doctors also gave Trump a steroid called dexamethasone to suppress his immune system, which was causing inflammation in his lungs. He was so ill that doctors considered sedating him and placing him on a ventilator—at which point Vice President Mike Pence would have taken over as commander in chief. Fortunately, Trump slowly improved. On October 5, 2020, three days after he had entered the hospital, Trump returned to the White House, certain that the monoclonal antibody Regeneron had saved his life.

Two years later, on July 21, 2022, President Joe Biden, who was 79 years old, tested positive for Covid. Because of his advanced age, Biden, like Trump, was at high risk for severe disease. Biden had already received four doses of mRNA vaccines. On the first day of his illness, he began taking an antiviral drug called Paxlovid. Whereas Trump had received his antiviral drug, remdesivir, intravenously, Biden took Paxlovid by mouth, suffering only a slight cough, runny nose, and mild fatigue. He continued to work at his desk in the White House. By July 26, five days after he had first tested positive for Covid, Biden's symptoms had largely resolved.

President Biden had one advantage over former President Trump in his fight against Covid: vaccines. Trump's illness began three months *before* Covid vaccines were available, Biden's 18 months *after* they had become available. And Trump didn't help himself by waiting until he had developed pneumonia. When he first developed symptoms, he could have taken the antiviral drug remdesivir or the monoclonal antibody preparation Regeneron, both of which would have decreased virus reproduction and prevented pneumonia. But Trump continued to deny his illness until he was severely ill. At that point, only the steroid dexamethasone, which lessened the inflammation in his lungs, could help. When Trump claimed that the monoclonal antibody preparation Regeneron had saved his life, he was wrong. If anything had saved his life, it was the dexamethasone.

WHICH COVID TREATMENTS
WORK BEST AT EACH STAGE?

The First (or Virus) Stage

President Biden was diagnosed during the first phase of Covid, when viral reproduction was central to the disease process. His treatment, therefore, was based on decreasing the ability of SARS-CoV-2 to reproduce itself. At this point, two possible strategies were available. One was antibodies that neutralized viruses *before* they had entered cells. The other was antiviral drugs that limited the capacity of viruses to reproduce themselves *after* they had entered cells.

We'll start with the antibodies.

Two types of antibody preparations are available to treat Covid during the early stage of illness: monoclonal antibodies and convalescent plasma. The FDA authorized the first monoclonal antibody cocktail (Regeneron) in November 2020. Many other monoclonal antibody products would soon follow. Before that, the only form of antibodies available was convalescent plasma.

The advantage of monoclonal antibodies is that they are synthesized in the laboratory and can therefore be used to treat millions of people. The disadvantage is that they recognize only one immunologically distinct region (called an epitope) on only one protein of the virus—specifically, the SARS-CoV-2 spike protein, which is responsible for attaching the virus to cells. Monoclonal antibodies are called monoclonal because they are the product of one B cell clone; therefore, they recognize only one epitope. Because SARS-CoV-2 is constantly changing, monoclonal antibodies that work against one variant might not work against another. For example, Regeneron, the monoclonal antibody cocktail that White House doctors had prescribed for President Trump, neutralized the viral variants circulating in 2020 but not the variant that infected President Biden two years later. Indeed, by the end of 2022, monoclonal antibodies didn't work against *any* of the circulating variants.

Convalescent plasma, on the other hand, contains antibodies that recognize many epitopes on all four SARS-CoV-2 viral proteins. Convalescent plasma is polyclonal (the product of many B cell clones), not monoclonal. Unfortunately, convalescent plasma depends on the generosity of people who have survived Covid and are willing to donate their blood. Also, convalescent plasma, which is administered intravenously, only works if it comes from people who make high quantities of high-quality antibodies to the virus; in other words, not all donated blood is valuable. But the good news about convalescent plasma is that, unlike monoclonal antibodies or possibly antivirals, it will never become obsolete as a weapon in the fight against Covid.

Although President Biden was diagnosed during the first phase of Covid, he didn't receive either monoclonal antibodies (which were available to treat the strain that had caused his infection) or convalescent plasma (which could have been obtained from blood donors who had been infected with the same strain). Rather, he was treated with the oral antiviral agent Paxlovid, which makes it much harder for the virus to reproduce itself. The advantage of Paxlovid is that it can be taken by mouth for about five days. President Biden took Paxlovid because of his age. In addition to the elderly, others who should also receive an antiviral drug during the first stage of illness are those who have compromised immunity or who have medical conditions that put them at high risk of suffering severe Covid.

When antivirals were first introduced, Paxlovid had the advantage over remdesivir in that it could be taken by mouth, whereas remdesivir is given intravenously. In December 2022, a preliminary study found that an oral preparation of remdesivir was as effective as Paxlovid in preventing Covid in high-risk, vaccinated participants. It is likely that oral remdesivir will eventually become available. Remdesivir has an advantage over Paxlovid, which interferes with other medications and can cause liver abnormalities. Also at the end of 2022, a study of high-risk patients in the United Kingdom found that molnupiravir, a different antiviral drug, was less effective than other antiviral drugs in preventing hospitalizations or deaths, making it the least effective antiviral.

Not everyone infected with Covid, however, needs to take antiviral therapies. Healthy young people who have been vaccinated don't need to receive monoclonal antibodies or antiviral drugs early in infection. When healthy people who have been vaccinated are exposed to SARS-CoV-2, they make antibodies quickly enough and in high enough quantities to prevent them from progressing to severe pneumonia.

The Second (or Immune) Stage

Ironically, our immune system works both for us and against us.

When SARS-CoV-2 enters our bodies and begins to reproduce itself, making millions of new virus particles, our immune system limits viral replication and spread. For people who are young and healthy, the immune system rids the body of SARS-CoV-2. When SARS-CoV-2 first entered the United States, the case fatality rate for children was .003 percent, meaning that 3 of every 100,000 children infected with Covid died from the disease. The case fatality rate for someone over 75, on the other hand, was about 3 percent, meaning that about 3 of every 100 elderly adults infected with Covid died from the disease. A thousandfold difference.

Of interest, the reason that people die from Covid is because their immune systems, while attempting to control the virus, can cause a lot of collateral damage. For example, lungs become flooded with immune cells, making it difficult to breathe, and occasionally requiring mechanical ventilation. Why does this happen? Why does our immune system eventually cause our death?

One possible explanation is that our immune system does everything possible to rid us of the virus—to a point. And when we reach the point where it looks like the virus is winning, our immune system, to prevent this deadly virus from spreading to others, culls us from the herd. At this stage, treatments that suppress the immune system provide the best chance for survival. This is what happened to President Trump, whose immune system caused his pneumonia; for that reason, doctors gave him dexamethasone, a steroid that calmed his immune system. However, drugs that suppress the immune system, when given during the first phase of illness, when the immune system is just starting to rid the body of the virus, can be quite harmful.

Given that neither monoclonal antibodies (like the Regeneron cocktail) nor antiviral drugs (like remdesivir) work in the second stage of illness, why did the doctors at Walter Reed National Military Hospital prescribe them for former President Trump? The FDA authorized remdesivir for treatment of Covid a few weeks after Trump became ill and Regeneron about one month after the start of his illness. At that point, clinicians had little experience with either of these two medications. It took time for studies to show that neither worked late in the illness.

Some people look at the story of Donald Trump and say, "See. That's why you can't trust doctors or scientists. They tell you one thing one day and something else the next."

But medical knowledge evolves over time. Fortunately, researchers are open-minded enough to know this, which is why Trump wouldn't have been treated with monoclonal antibodies or antiviral

drugs in 2022. The circumspection and fluidity of science and medicine, though disconcerting to some, are exactly why people should
trust the scientific process. Doctors and scientists aren't so rigid that
they ignore new evidence.

WHICH COVID TREATMENTS SHOULD BE AVOIDED?

Four medicines that are often used to treat Covid should be avoided.

Steroids

Steroids like dexamethasone suppress the immune system. Therefore, late in Covid infections, when the immune system is doing more
harm than good, steroids can be lifesaving. Early in Covid, however,
when the immune system is doing what it can to limit viral reproduction, steroids can be quite harmful. Indeed, in October 2020, the
National Institutes of Health issued guidelines restricting steroid use
only to those patients who required oxygen for severe pneumonia.

In 2022, researchers from the FDA, the Department of Veterans
Affairs, and Harvard Medical School studied two large health care
databases to determine whether steroids were being used appropri-
ately. They found that by August 2021, after the guidelines for steroid
use had been clearly established and communicated for almost a year,
about 20 percent of Medicare patients seen as outpatients with Covid
had received steroids early in their illness. Suppressing the immune
system during the first stage of illness in patients trying to survive
Covid is arguably the single most dangerous thing a doctor can do
while trying to treat this disease. Timing is everything.

Hydroxychloroquine

In 2020, before we had vaccines, monoclonal antibodies, or antiviral
agents, people were hoping that other drugs sitting on a pharmacist's

shelf might also work to treat Covid. These were called "repurposed drugs." Hydroxychloroquine and ivermectin are two examples.

Hydroxychloroquine is a drug used to treat malaria. In chapter 3, we described three large studies that showed that hydroxychloroquine not only didn't treat or prevent Covid but could cause heart arrhythmias, a potentially fatal side effect. Given those studies, why do some patients continue to demand it and some doctors continue to prescribe it? In part, this is a result of promotion of the drug by anti-vaccine activists who hold firmly to the notion that we don't need vaccines if easy-to-obtain drugs like hydroxychloroquine are available.

Ivermectin

Ivermectin, which was discovered in 1975, is used by veterinarians to treat horses infected with parasites such as heartworm and roundworm. Before SARS-CoV-2 entered the United States, researchers had also tested ivermectin against a variety of different viruses in the hopes it would work. It didn't.

In March 2022, 490 people with Covid were randomly divided into two groups; 241 were given ivermectin and 249 were given a placebo pill. Investigators found that 22 percent of people who had received ivermectin developed severe disease, compared with 17 percent in the placebo group. No differences were observed between the groups in the need for intensive care support or mechanical ventilation. And the death rate was the same. The only difference was that people who received ivermectin were more likely to have diarrhea, headaches, muscle aches, dizziness, nausea, and a skin rash.

Activists refused to believe the results of this study, arguing that researchers needed to use a higher dose of ivermectin. In response, one year later, in March 2023, researchers divided 1,200 patients with

Covid into two groups. One received high-dose ivermectin; the other didn't. The results were the same: No differences were observed in time to sustained recovery from Covid in those who received ivermectin.

The futility of ivermectin as a treatment for Covid, the promotion of the drug by Robert Malone on Joe Rogan's podcast, the fact that many people took ivermectin while at the same time refusing vaccines, and the origins of the drug as a treatment for horses inspired several humorous memes and videos with taglines such as, "Just say neigh to ivermectin," and "Ask your large animal veterinarian whether ivermectin is right for you."

As late as May 2022, well after both hydroxychloroquine and ivermectin had been shown to be ineffective, Republicans in several states, including New Hampshire, Tennessee, Ohio, and Kansas, introduced legislation to allow physicians greater freedom to prescribe these useless, non-FDA approved, potentially dangerous drugs. The legislation also protected the doctors who prescribed them from administrative discipline and civil litigation.

Antibiotics

Antibiotics treat bacterial infections, not viral infections. Nonetheless, in May 2022, researchers from the CDC found that 30 percent of people with Covid had received a prescription for an antibiotic. Antibiotics, like all medicines, can cause serious side effects, including allergic reactions.

WHAT COVID TREATMENTS ARE LIKELY TO BE AVAILABLE IN THE FUTURE?

When SARS-CoV-2 entered the United States in January 2020, little was available to treat or prevent it. Other than masking, social distancing, testing, isolating, and quarantining, the only way to curb the devastation of Covid was with convalescent plasma.

But within two years, major strides had been made. We had oral antiviral medicines that could be taken easily and worked well in people who were at high risk of severe Covid. We had long-acting monoclonal antibodies that could prevent severe disease for months in high-risk patients. And we had vaccines that were effective, widely available, and free of charge.

Given the pace of innovation in the first three years, it is reasonable to assume that therapies will continue to evolve. What does the future hold for the treatment of Covid?

Antivirals

At the end of 2022, Paxlovid, which reduced the incidence of severe disease by as much as 90 percent, was the antiviral drug of choice for people early in their illness who were immune compromised, elderly, or had high-risk conditions such as obesity, or chronic heart, lung, or kidney disease. Paxlovid was much more effective than the other antiviral drug that was taken by mouth, molnupiravir, and had an advantage over remdesivir, which had to be administered intravenously.

By late 2022, however, preliminary studies showed that an oral form of remdesivir, which was still in the experimental stage, worked just as well as Paxlovid. Also, remdesivir, unlike Paxlovid, doesn't interact with other medications. It is likely that new antiviral medicines will become available during the next decade. It is also possible that, in a manner identical to the antiviral medications used to treat HIV and hepatitis C virus, combination drugs might be found to be more effective than stand-alone, single treatments.

Despite its remarkable effectiveness in treating Covid in high-risk groups, Paxlovid has suffered from the common misconception that it causes "Paxlovid rebound," which has been reported to occur in 3 to 5 percent of people taking the drug. Paxlovid rebound is defined as an increase in Covid symptoms soon after stopping the drug. The implication is that once the antiviral drug is stopped, the virus is once again free to reproduce itself and cause symptoms. But that's not what's happening.

Again, we need to divide Covid into two phases: In the first phase, virus replication is king; in the second phase, the immune response, which is what causes symptoms, is king. However, late in the first phase of illness, after the treatment course of Paxlovid has been completed, the immune system's response to the viral infection becomes more vigorous, causing an increase in symptoms. So, the "rebound" isn't caused by a "freeing" of the virus after stopping the drug; it's caused by the immune system starting to exert an effect.

Indeed, the incidence of "rebound" in people with Covid is the same in people who did or didn't take Paxlovid—so more accurately, the phenomenon should be called "Covid rebound." For that reason, people don't need to restart the drug; at that point, it's too late for Paxlovid to make a difference, because we've moved from the viral replication stage into the beginning of the immune response stage.

Monoclonal Antibodies

In November 2020, the FDA authorized Regeneron for the treatment of Covid. The generic names of the two monoclonal preparations in the drug were casirivimab and imdevimab. (The generic names of monoclonal antibodies are invariably unpronounceable.)

Regeneron worked well against the variants that circulated in the United States in 2021, such as Alpha and Delta. But when Omicron (BA.1) and the Omicron subvariants (BA.2, BA.3, BA.4, and BA.5) made their debut in early 2022, it became obsolete; Omicron and its subvariants had changed so much that antibodies in Regeneron no longer recognized the virus. This was also true for many other monoclonal antibody preparations that had come on the market, all with similarly unpronounceable generic names like bebtelovimab, bamlanivimab, etesevimab, casirivimab, imdevimab, sotrovimab, and a combination product that contained tixagevimab and cilgavimab (Evusheld). (The names of all monoclonal antibodies end in "-mab.") By the end of 2022, all commercially available preparations of monoclonal antibodies had become ineffective.

The future of monoclonal antibodies as a treatment for the first stage of Covid remains uncertain. One new broadly reacting monoclonal antibody called adintrevimab, first reported in March 2023, has shown some promise. Time will tell. However, as variants continue to evolve, it's understandable that pharmaceutical companies wouldn't make an investment on a product that might soon become obsolete.

Convalescent Plasma

Convalescent plasma has once again become important in our war against SARS-CoV-2. A study published in 2022 found that convalescent plasma obtained from people who had survived Covid reduced the risk of hospitalization by 54 percent in those who had been treated within eight days of the onset of symptoms. All the participants in this study were unvaccinated.

At the beginning of 2023, no group benefited more from convalescent plasma than immune-compromised people who couldn't be effectively vaccinated. In this group, monoclonal antibodies had been the only way to prevent illness. When monoclonal antibodies became obsolete at the end of 2022, the only way to prevent illness in this group was with convalescent plasma, which was not readily available.

Convalescent plasma might eventually become an important tool for all high-risk groups if, in the worst-case scenario, a variant of

SARS-CoV-2 evolves to become completely resistant to vaccines and antiviral drugs. Convalescent plasma would be a useful tool during the time it would take to make a new vaccine to prevent this novel variant.

Immune-Suppressive Drugs

Steroids, such as dexamethasone, are powerful immunosuppressive agents. But they're not very specific, suppressing virtually every aspect of the immune system. Steroids prevent B cells from making antibodies, T cells from helping B cells make antibodies, and cytotoxic T cells from killing virus-infected cells. They also suppress white blood cells called neutrophils from killing bacteria. For this reason, people receiving steroids are at high risk of being overwhelmed by a variety of different infections.

It is likely that we will get better at suppressing the immune system more specifically in the years to come; indeed, it's already happening. For example, "cytokine storm" is a massive and occasionally fatal inflammation of the lungs triggered by Covid. (Cytokines are products of the immune system and include a variety of interleukins and interferons.) Cytokine storm is typically caused by the overproduction of one specific immune protein called interleukin-6, or IL-6. A monoclonal antibody preparation aimed at neutralizing the effects of IL-6 (called tocilizumab) is now commercially available. It has become a mainstay in treating patients with Covid who suffer cytokine storm.

As we get better at defining the immunological proteins causing severe Covid, we will likely get better at targeting specific components of the immune system that are responsible for causing harm.

CHAPTER 10

LONG COVID: WHAT IS IT? CAN IT BE TREATED? CAN IT BE PREVENTED?

- What is long Covid?
- What causes long Covid?
- Can long Covid be treated?
- Why is long Covid controversial?
- What are the best ways to avoid long Covid?

In 2020, when our hospital—the Children's Hospital of Philadelphia—was overflowing with Covid patients, I saw children suffering from something I had never seen before. Their stories were eerily similar. All were between five and 13 years of age, and all had mild symptoms like congestion, cough, or runny nose that resolved quickly. Their infection apparently behind them, these children ran and played, ate normally, and went back to school.

One month later, however, they developed high fever, shaking chills, rashes, abdominal pain, vomiting, breathing difficulties, neurological dysfunction, and heart, liver, and kidney damage. Several went to the intensive care unit, taking weeks and sometimes months to fully recover. Their disease was called multisystem inflammatory syndrome in children, or MIS-C. By the end of December 2022, about 9,000 children in the United States had suffered from MIS-C, and 76 had died. Worse, MIS-C wasn't limited to children; the adult form was called multisystem inflammatory syndrome in adults (MIS-A).

The phenomenon of long-lasting symptoms wasn't unique to Covid. Viruses such as influenza, Ebola, HIV, hepatitis B, hepatitis C, Epstein-Barr virus (the cause of mono), and others can also cause long-term symptoms. What was unique about MIS-C was that these long-lasting symptoms occurred after what appeared to have been a complete resolution of the disease.

WHAT IS LONG COVID?

The term "long Covid" became popular with the widespread use of #LongCovid on Twitter. The symptoms of long Covid, which read like the index of a medical textbook, involve every major organ system.

Long Covid affects the lungs, causing breathlessness, persistent cough, worsening of asthma, chest pain, and impaired exercise capacity. More than half of patients with long Covid have abnormal chest x-rays.

Long Covid also affects the heart, causing palpitations, slow or rapid heartbeats, chest pain, chest tightness, arrhythmias, low blood pressure, fainting, and heart enlargement. Most of these patients have abnormal heart scans or electrocardiograms (EKGs). Further evidence of heart damage is seen when an enzyme found in heart muscle cells called troponin spills into the bloodstream.

Long Covid also affects the intestinal tract, liver, and pancreas, causing loss of appetite, abdominal pain, nausea, vomiting, weight loss, irritable bowel syndrome, and difficulty swallowing. Like damage to the heart, evidence of damage to the liver and pancreas is seen when enzymes specific to those organs are detected in the bloodstream.

Long Covid can also affect the muscles, bones, and joints, causing weakness, joint pain, and arthritis.

Most commonly, long Covid causes general symptoms such as fatigue, poor concentration, restriction of daily activities, malaise, and weakness, all of which can worsen following even small amounts of physical or mental exertion. For some, including previously fit, athletic people who regularly climbed mountains and ran marathons, even showering or brushing teeth can leave them exhausted and bedridden.

Long Covid is also accompanied by a daunting list of laboratory abnormalities, including elevated white blood cells, anemia, lipid abnormalities, elevated hemoglobin A1C (a marker for prediabetes), reduced serum albumin (a protein made in the liver), low platelets (cells in the bloodstream necessary for clotting), other clotting abnormalities, and disturbances in electrolytes such as sodium and potassium.

But the most debilitating symptoms of long Covid, which ironically have caused the most controversy, are those involving the brain. Symptoms include disturbed sleep, loss of taste and smell for more than two months, mood swings, depression, stress, anxiety, numbness and tingling in the fingers, tinnitus (ringing in the ears), feeling alternatively hot and cold, seizures, headaches, dizziness, blurred vision, defects in memory and concentration, hallucinations, psychosis, tremor, and, finally, brain fog, which is the inability to concentrate or to think clearly, as well as difficulty remembering things. Objective evidence of brain involvement can be found in imaging studies of the brain, showing destruction of the olfactory bulb, which is responsible for the sense of smell. Some researchers have also detected SARS-CoV-2 in the brain in autopsy studies. Others have detected destruction of blood vessels supplying oxygen to the brain or evidence for brain inflammation.

Although long Covid is defined as symptoms lasting more than four weeks, they can last much longer. About 70 percent of those affected have symptoms lasting for 12 weeks, 40 percent for at least a year, and 20 percent for at least two years. The most common symptoms are fatigue (87 percent), malaise (83 percent), brain fog (81 percent), sleep disorders (77 percent), and lethargy (75 percent).

WHAT CAUSES LONG COVID?

Clues to the cause or causes of long Covid can be found in the fact that it affects the lungs, heart, kidneys, liver, skin, intestines, muscles, bones, spleen, and brain. What do all these organs have in common? A blood supply. SARS-CoV-2 affects the blood vessels that supply oxygen to each of these organs. Deprived of oxygen, these organs can become dysfunctional.

Three possible mechanisms have been offered to explain what causes long Covid, all of which are overlapping and none of which are mutually exclusive.

The first possible explanation is that SARS-CoV-2 is continuing to reproduce itself for weeks or months, much longer than other respiratory viruses. In support of this theory, researchers at the National Institutes of Health performed autopsies on 44 people who died from Covid. They found that SARS-CoV-2 was reproducing itself in a wide variety of organs, including the brain, muscles, intestines, and lungs. Although most of these autopsies were performed on people who had died from Covid, five were performed on people who had mild or asymptomatic Covid and had died from something else. If this mechanism is found to best explain the cause of long Covid, then antiviral medications might be of value. Time and further study will likely answer this question.

The second possible explanation is that SARS-CoV-2 causes persistent activation of the immune system, even after the virus has been eliminated from the body. In support of this theory, researchers at the Icahn School of Medicine in New York found that immune cells in patients with long Covid continued to be activated eight months after infection. They also found that certain proteins (called interferons) produced by the immune system predicted long Covid with 80 percent accuracy. This suggested either a delayed or defective resolution of the immune response in patients with long Covid. If this mechanism is found to best explain the cause of long Covid, then drugs that suppress the immune system broadly, such as steroids, or more specifically, such as monoclonal antibodies directed against immune proteins, might be of value. Because immuno-suppressive therapies can have dangerous side effects, it would be important to prove that they work before recommending them. Again, time will tell.

The third possible explanation is that SARS-CoV-2 causes small clots that can block blood vessels. During acute infection, small blood clots have been detected in the lungs, as well as in a variety of other organs. These blood clots can persist for months or even years. If this is the case, then medications that melt clots would be of value. These medications also carry significant risks.

The story of one 14-year-old girl in Rome shows how these different possible causes of long Covid can be overlapping. In October 2020, the girl suffered low-grade fever, runny nose, and loss of taste and smell. Before Covid, she was playful and active, riding horses and playing music. She had no other medical problems. Thirty days after the start of her illness, however, and well after her symptoms had completely resolved, she developed head-ache, chest pain, fatigue, and a rapid heart rate. In May 2021, seven months after symptoms of long Covid had begun, she was admitted to the hospital. Doctors found that she had the exact same immu-nological abnormalities that researchers at the Icahn School of Medicine in New York had described, as well as small blood clots located throughout her lungs. The doctors treated her with ste-roids to suppress her immune system and heparin to dissolve the blood clots. The plan was to treat her for six to nine months. "The biggest obstacle we are facing [with long Covid] is that we gave it one name. We gave it the name of long Covid, which implies that it is one disease" says Chahinda Ghossein, a physician and heart disease researcher at Maastricht University in the Netherlands. "All the studies being performed show us that it is not." Several studies are now in progress across the globe to determine the value of antiviral medicines, immunosuppressive therapies, and clot-dissolving medicines alone or in combination to treat long Covid.

CAN LONG COVID BE TREATED?

A few simpler therapies have already been shown to be effective. Researchers in China found that aerobic exercises, balance training, breathing training, and resistance/strength training twice a day for at least 30 minutes each day dramatically lessened the incidence of long-term symptoms, including fatigue, headache, anxiety, lung dysfunction, malaise, and lethargy, for people with Covid recently discharged from the hospital.

Unfortunately, for disorders like long Covid, for which no defin-itive diagnostic test or treatment exists, the internet often steps in, offering a wide range of can't-miss cures such as antibiotics, vitamin C, hydroxychloroquine, nutritional and dietary supplements, and antiretroviral medicines (such as those used to treat AIDS patients). Those afflicted with long Covid should beware of these false claims. When so many supplements are all touted as working, healthy skepticism should rule, at the very least because many of these therapies are costly and some are harmful.

WHY IS LONG COVID CONTROVERSIAL?

Many people suffering from long Covid have objective, verifiable, laboratory-confirmed damage to different organs. As of April 2023, the CDC estimated that at least 26 million Americans were suffering from this disease; four million Americans—about 2.4 percent of the workforce—had to leave their full-time jobs.

Moreover, long Covid isn't unique to the United States; hundreds of millions of people across the globe have been affected. At least 90 advocacy groups fighting for more research, improved treatments, and increased access to disability benefits have sprung up in 34 countries. Of interest, long Covid isn't unique to the SARS-CoV-2 coronavirus; it was also seen following infections with the coronaviruses SARS-CoV-1 and MERS, with some symptoms lasting up to 15 years.

Those suffering from long Covid feel abandoned, ignored, or worse, labeled as malingerers and cranks. Why?

One possible explanation is that the most common symptoms of long Covid are fatigue, brain fog, sleep disorders, lethargy, muscle pain, and malaise. Although it is easy to determine whether the lung is damaged with a chest x-ray or whether the heart is damaged with an EKG, it is much harder to measure fatigue, muscle pain, malaise, or brain fog, which are subjective. Fatigue and pain are whatever the patient says they are.

Another problem with long Covid is defining it. Studies of the disease have described long Covid as persistent symptoms lasting for either four, eight, or 12 weeks from the start of the illness. It's important to determine whether symptoms are just a prolonged recovery from initial damage to various organs, or the product of a hyperactive immune system, persistent viral replication, or uncontrolled blood clotting occurring after the acute illness has resolved.

Despite public awareness of long Covid, many who suffer the disease feel abandoned. "We are just left to rot," said Chantal Britt, founder and president of Long Covid Switzerland. "That's why all these organizations are popping up," said Jo House, a long Covid advocate in the United Kingdom. "There is no official help. Increasingly, the governments just want to move on. Everything is about, 'We must live with Covid now.' There isn't the same sense of urgency, which is tragic given the vast number of people ill with this."

Doctors are also frustrated. "There are so many things that we need to learn, and no one is helping us," said Eleni Iasonidou, a pediatrician who heads Long Covid Greece. "In 10 years from now, we will have answers and long Covid will take its place as a disease. But in the meantime, we're all here and we must live with that."

The perception of long Covid is also influenced by the way in which it first came to public attention. Awareness of this extended form of the disease was born of people suffering from it—first on Twitter, and then in patient support groups like Body Politic, which launched in 2018 and described itself as a "wellness collective merging the personal and the political." Two years later, in March 2020, the group created the Body Politic Covid-19 support group, as part of its mission to create "patient-led research." If scientists and doctors weren't going to study this disease, then patients would do it themselves.

Unfortunately, many of those who responded to Body Politic's initial survey probably never had Covid. Of those who self-identified as having long Covid, fewer than 25 percent had tested positive for the virus, about half had never been tested, and 25 percent had tested negative. When Body Politic did a follow-up survey in December 2020, one year into the pandemic, only 600 (about 16 percent) of the 3,800 respondents had ever tested positive for the virus.

Another possible explanation for difficulties appreciating long Covid as a separate entity is that it might be a different illness, at least for some people. Because the prominent symptoms of long Covid are fatigue, sleeplessness, malaise, lethargy, and brain fog, it's important to distinguish long Covid from clinical depression, which might be more a consequence of the measures put in place to stop the spread of the virus than the virus itself. Several studies have shown that the longer a person is isolated or quarantined, the poorer the mental health outcomes. Indeed, in one prospective, well-controlled, multicenter study published in 2022, participants who suffered from poor physical, mental, or social well-being for three months following a respiratory illness were tested to see if they had had Covid. Two-thirds had. But a third hadn't, presumably suffering the isolation and severe restrictions put in place during the pandemic.

It is also possible that some diseases attributed to Covid are a product of a disrupted health care system and not the virus. For example, researchers in Germany, studying more than 5,000 children and adolescents, found a dramatic increase in the incidence of type 1 diabetes. Researchers at the CDC also found a rise in type 1 diabetes in the United States during the pandemic. The implication was that type 1 diabetes was a long-term consequence of Covid. However, after examining the records of more than two million children, researchers in Ontario, Canada, found no such increase, arguing that the dramatic rise of type 1 diabetes in the other studies could be explained by a rapid return to the health care system after isolation and quarantining had lightened. Time will tell whether Covid is a cause of type 1 diabetes.

Finally, in 2022, with increasing awareness of long Covid, researchers in the state of Georgia found a discrepancy between self-reported problems and objective confirmation of those problems. About 50 percent of those claiming long Covid reported a loss of taste or smell that wasn't confirmed on objective tests. Similarly, patients who reported symptoms such as confusion and brain fog were not more likely to have deficits on quantitative cognitive testing when compared with those who had never reported those symptoms.

One thing, however, is clear: Long Covid is both real and devastating. Finding a way to treat and prevent it will be just as important as preventing Covid hospitalizations. "The two diseases—acute Covid and long Covid—aren't very different," says David Lee, an emergency medicine doctor at New York University School of Medicine.

WHAT ARE THE BEST WAYS TO AVOID LONG COVID?

For many through this pandemic, there is no greater fear than that of long Covid. The notion that people would have to suffer debilitating symptoms for weeks, months, or even years following Covid infection has driven many into the waiting arms of the alternative medicine industry and a coven of quack physicians. The good news is that people can do three things to lessen the risk of long Covid.

First, get vaccinated. Researchers in the United Kingdom studied more than a million people with Covid to determine whether vaccination reduced the incidence of symptoms lasting more than a month. They found that those who had received at least two doses of vaccine were significantly less likely to develop long Covid. Similarly, a study performed in the United States during the Omicron variant outbreak found that vaccination reduced the incidence of long Covid by about 50 percent. Finally, researchers in Italy found that 42 percent of people with Covid who developed long Covid were unvaccinated. For those who had received one dose of vaccine prior to getting Covid, the incidence of long Covid was 30 percent; for those who had received two doses, it was 17 percent; and for those who had received three doses, it was 16 percent. Presumably, those who had been vaccinated against Covid had a lesser burden of virus, and therefore a lesser chance of developing long Covid, than those who were unvaccinated. But, at least in this Italian study, the incidence of long Covid didn't lessen with booster doses.

Second, reduce your chance of being infected. This won't be easy. But some practical strategies make sense. If you are in a crowded public place indoors, and you are worried about long Covid, wear a mask, especially during the winter months. High-quality (not cloth) masks, particularly well-fitting N95 or KN95 masks, are highly effective at lessening the risk of contact with the virus. They don't eliminate the risk, but they clearly decrease it.

Because people are less likely to be infected with SARS-CoV-2 if they are outdoors, another way to reduce your chance of being infected is to increase the amount of outdoor air coming inside. Opening windows and doors, turning on window or attic fans, running a window air conditioner with the vent control open, and operating kitchen or bathroom fans that exhaust air outdoors all increase ventilation and lessen the spread of viruses. In addition to ventilation, air filtration systems lessen the spread of viruses by directly removing viral particles from the air. In the home, portable air cleaners that remove particles as small as 0.3 micrometer effectively decrease the concentration of viruses in the air. Outside the home, most schools, offices, and businesses with heating, ventilation, and air conditioning (HVAC) systems have filters that remove small particles. Crowded, poorly ventilated rooms without an HVAC system should be avoided.

Finally, if you are in a high-risk group, make sure to take an antiviral drug early in illness, which like vaccination, may decrease the chance of long Covid.

BY THE BEGINNING OF 2023, after SARS-CoV-2 had been circulating in the United States for about three years, millions of people had suffered from long Covid. Given that the virus is likely to circulate for decades, these numbers will only increase. To put this in perspective, every year in the United States about two million people are diagnosed with cancer and 1.5 million with diabetes. Those suffering from long Covid will likely eclipse these numbers for many years to come.

The care and treatment of long Covid has fallen to the health care system, which will be responsible for developing diagnostic criteria and effective treatments. Who will pay for all this care? The avalanche of disability insurance claims will fall to both public and private employers. For private health insurers, increased costs will be passed on to employers. For public health insurers, state and federal governments will bear the cost. Those who are self-employed or work in small businesses, which often offer no insurance benefits, will cause a disparity in treatments. As is true in many aspects of the health care system, these disparities will cause differences in care among the rich and poor.

Some good news: The incidence of long Covid appears to be declining. In March 2023, a study reported in the *British Journal of*

Haematology found that the risk of long Covid symptoms three months after infection had dropped from 46 percent with the original Wuhan-1 strain to 35 percent with the Delta variant to 14 percent with the Omicron variant.

As we learn more about how to diagnose and treat long Covid, it's likely that the impact of this surprising and devastating problem will only continue to decline.

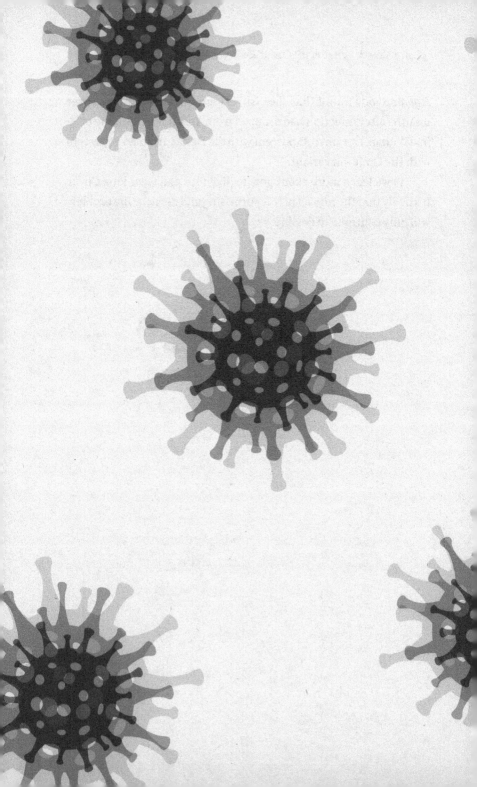

PART III

WHERE WE'RE HEADING

CHAPTER 11

CAN WE MAKE A BETTER COVID VACCINE?

- Can we make a Covid vaccine that provides long-lived protection against mild disease?
- Can we make a Covid vaccine for people who fear needles?
- Can we make a Covid vaccine that is variant-proof?
- Can we make a Covid vaccine that protects against all future coronavirus pandemics?

On July 26, 2022, President Joe Biden hosted the "White House Summit on the Future of Covid-19 Vaccines." Dr. Ashish Jha, the White House's Covid response coordinator, introduced the program. "The vaccines we have are terrific," he said. "But we can do better than terrific." The question is: Can we?

CAN WE MAKE A COVID VACCINE THAT PROVIDES LONG-LIVED PROTECTION AGAINST MILD DISEASE?

The mRNA vaccines made by Pfizer and Moderna, the viral vector vaccines made by Johnson & Johnson, and the purified protein vaccine made by Novavax all offer a high level of protection against mild illness. But not for long. Several months after the last dose of these vaccines, protection against mild illness fades.

Enter nasal spray vaccines.

SARS-CoV-2 initially reproduces itself in the lining of the nose and throat. Wouldn't it make sense, then, to find a way to induce a vigorous, active immune response at the site where the virus enters the body as a first line of defense—a way to provide better, longer-lasting protection against mild illness and to decrease transmission? "We're stopping the virus from spreading right at the border," said Akiko Iwasaki, an immunologist at Yale University who is working on nasal spray vaccines. "This is akin to putting a guard outside of the house in order to patrol for invaders compared to putting the guards in the hallway of the building in the hope that they capture the invader." It's also much easier to give and receive a nasal spray vaccine than a shot—and sometimes, much cheaper.

As this book was being written, many possible strategies to make a nasal spray vaccine had been tested in animal models such as mice, monkeys, ferrets, and hamsters, often with exciting results. Researchers have inoculated animals with nasal sprays containing mRNA vaccines, purified protein vaccines, viral vector vaccines, or live, weakened forms of SARS-CoV-2 (like the vaccines currently given as shots to prevent measles, mumps, and chicken pox). Some of these nasal spray vaccines have now advanced to studies in people.

Speaking at the White House Summit hosted by Jha, Marty Moore, the chief executive officer for a California-based company called Meissa Vaccines, observed, "No one here today can tell you that [nasal spray] vaccines work; we're not there yet. We need clinical efficacy data to answer that question." Nonetheless, Moore believes that nasal spray vaccines have the potential to deliver "a knockout blow to Covid" and serve as a "transmission-blocking machine."

Caution, however, should reign. Nasal spray vaccines and vaccines given as a shot induce different kinds of antibodies. Vaccines given as shots induce immunoglobulin G (IgG), which hangs out in the bloodstream, not on the lining of the nose or throat. Nasal spray vaccines, in addition to IgG, also induce immunoglobulin A (IgA), which resides on mucosal surfaces such as the lining of the nose, throat, and intestines. The good news about IgA is that it can withstand the harsh environment of mucosal surfaces. The bad news is that IgA induced at mucosal surfaces, like IgG in the bloodstream, is short-lived. A few months after an intranasal vaccine, virus-specific IgA will also begin to fade away.

Researchers working on nasal spray vaccines argue that although they understand antibodies on the lining of the nose and throat are short-lived, memory immune cells are long-lived. And these memory cells, which would now reside under the lining of the nose, would be poised to spring into action when the body encounters the virus. Unfortunately, like memory cells induced in the body after a Covid vaccine shot, memory cells induced in the nasal mucosa also take several days to become activated. For that reason, even the world's best nasal spray vaccine won't make much of a dent on mild illness, viral shedding, or viral transmission for very long after vaccination. Indeed, FluMist, a nasal spray vaccine to prevent influenza, which has been available since 2003, has been far from a game changer, failing to provide better or longer-lasting protection against mild infections than influenza vaccines given as shots.

Nasal spray vaccines will likely offer some benefit in preventing mild infection and transmission above vaccines given as a shot—at least for several months. But we will never be able to prevent mild Covid illness for long because the incubation period of the virus is short (see chapter 8). And nothing can be done to lengthen the incubation period of the infection. Quite the opposite: Since we have progressed from the Alpha to Delta to Omicron variants, incubation periods have only grown shorter.

CAN WE MAKE A COVID VACCINE FOR PEOPLE WHO FEAR NEEDLES?

One advantage of nasal spray vaccines is something that most people don't like to talk about: needle phobia. On April 10, 2021, Rachel Maddow shared her experience in this arena with millions of her viewers on MSNBC. "I'm afraid of needles," said Maddow, describing how she shed tears of gratitude after surviving her first vaccination. "We need to understand these fears, which are reasonable. It's nothing to be ashamed of."

Needle phobia isn't as rare as one might imagine. Before the Covid pandemic, researchers found that the phenomenon affected 25 percent of adults and likely caused 16 percent to skip or delay vaccines. During the Covid pandemic, 14 percent of people who chose not to be vaccinated cited fear of needles as the reason. This is not a trivial anxiety; the condition causes hyperventilation, fainting, and panic attacks.

Although no program in the United States addresses this problem, national health programs in Canada and the United Kingdom do. Adults who say they are afraid of needles aren't vaccinated in public; instead, they are taken to a private room to receive their vaccines. Clinicians find that it helps to say the fear out loud. But the unending images on television and the internet of people wincing while getting jabbed isn't helping.

In addition to nasal spray vaccines, micropatch vaccines offer another way to avoid needle phobia. These dime-size patches consist of 100 water-soluble needles that contain the vaccine. The tiny needles, which barely penetrate the skin, dissolve in minutes. Micropatch technology, which is now decades old, could be used to prevent Covid and solve the problem of needle phobia. Unfortunately, pharmaceutical companies (at least to this point) aren't convinced that people with needle phobia make up a large enough percentage of the population to make micropatch vaccines commercially viable. Which is too bad, because micropatch technology could also be used to vaccinate children, virtually all of whom fear needles.

CAN WE MAKE A COVID VACCINE THAT IS VARIANT-PROOF?

To date, all SARS-CoV-2 variants have been recognized by T cells (see chapter 8). That's why the original Wuhan-1 vaccines have continued to provide protection against severe disease for the Alpha, Delta, and Omicron variants. If, however, a variant arises that escapes recognition by T cells induced by vaccination or previous infection, then we will need to reimmunize the entire population to protect against this new variant.

It is likely that vaccines containing the Wuhan-1 strain, which at the beginning of 2023 was present in the bivalent vaccine, will become obsolete, only to be replaced by yearly monovalent, bivalent, or multivalent vaccines that contain the current circulating strains in much the same manner as yearly influenza vaccines. Indeed, in June 2023, the CDC recommended that Covid vaccines contain only one of the circulating Omicron strains, eliminating the Wuhan-1 strain from the vaccine.

CAN WE MAKE A COVID VACCINE THAT PROTECTS AGAINST ALL FUTURE CORONAVIRUS PANDEMICS?

Wouldn't it be nice to have a vaccine that protects against not only SARS-CoV-2 but all coronaviruses with the potential to cause a pandemic? One that protects against viruses like SARS-CoV-1 (which caused an outbreak in 2003), MERS (which caused an outbreak in 2012), as well as all the other coronaviruses now circulating in bats and other small mammals lurking in caves and forests throughout the world? How hard could that be? Turns out, very hard.

As an explanation, I offer two, true-life cautionary tales: one, a universal influenza vaccine that eliminates the need for yearly dosing, and the other, an HIV vaccine to prevent AIDS.

Influenza virus is composed of 11 proteins. (SARS-CoV-2 is composed of four proteins). The most important influenza virus protein, which attaches the virus to cells, is called the hemagglutinin, or HA, protein. The reason we need a yearly influenza vaccine is that the HA protein changes. Indeed, it changes so much from one year to the next that immunization or natural infection the previous year might not protect against severe disease the following year. (The HA can also change during a single winter season, which is why the influenza vaccine is only about 60 percent effective in protecting against severe disease.)

Although the HA protein from influenza is constantly changing, many regions on the other influenza proteins don't change much; they remain relatively constant for *all* influenza strains. In fact, several regions on the HA protein also remain relatively constant. So, wouldn't it make sense to make a vaccine that includes those conserved regions—the ones that don't seem to change very much? Then we wouldn't need a yearly vaccine; we would be protected against all influenza strains.

Researchers have been trying to do exactly that for the last 50 years. But, as it turns out, it's much easier said than done. We are no closer now to a universal influenza vaccine than we were 50 years ago. (In the 1980s, I trained in a laboratory that studied influenza virus. The head of that laboratory, Dr. Walter Gerhard, once said something to me that I'll never forget: "If you want a research career that lasts for the rest of your life," he said, "study influenza.")

Attempts to make an HIV vaccine, which began in the early 1980s, further exemplify the difficulties of making a universal coronavirus vaccine. People who are infected with HIV rapidly make antibodies that neutralize the virus; those antibodies work well to eliminate the infecting strain. The problem with HIV is that the virus constantly changes *during a single infection;* antibodies that work at the beginning of the illness don't work at all as the illness progresses and the virus continues to evolve. HIV is the ultimate moving target.

The good news is that HIV, like influenza and SARS-CoV-2, has many regions on its 15 proteins that are highly conserved, and these regions don't change during infection. Companies have now spent billions of dollars trying to make vaccines directed against these highly conserved regions—again, like attempts to make a universal influenza vaccine, without success. And it's not for lack of money, expertise, or hard work: Efforts to make universal influenza and HIV vaccines have received billions of dollars in funding over the last few decades.

In 2021, researchers around the globe began publishing exciting results about vaccines that could protect against all future pandemic coronaviruses (called pan-sarbecovirus vaccines). These studies were performed in animal models and were met with a level of excitement similar to early studies on universal influenza or HIV vaccines, which were also performed in animal models.

Protection against disease in animals, however, doesn't always predict protection against disease in people. Therefore, our experiences with influenza and HIV vaccines should serve as cautionary tales about the likelihood that a vaccine will work against all possible strains of coronavirus.

But you never know.

ON APRIL 10, 2023, the White House announced the creation of a $5 billion program intended in part to create newer, better coronavirus vaccines. Focusing on nasal spray vaccines and universal coronavirus vaccines, the program was called "Project NextGen." "It's been very clear to us that the market on this is moving very slowly," said White House Covid response coordinator Ashish Jha. "There's a lot that government can do, the administration can do, to speed up those tools ... for the American people."

CHAPTER 12

SHOULD COVID VACCINES BE MANDATED?

- Are vaccine mandates constitutional?
- Can states legally mandate vaccines for school entry?
- Should Covid vaccines be mandated post-pandemic?

Throughout 2020, the only way to stop the spread of SARS-CoV-2 was by preventing people from interacting with one another. We masked, social distanced, isolated, quarantined, shut down businesses, closed schools, restricted travel, and tested, tested, tested. It was all we could do.

Then, in December 2020, two vaccines were offered to the American public free of charge. Millions rushed to get them. Many, however, chose to remain unprotected. What to do? Here were people who, claiming personal freedoms, civil liberties, and bodily autonomy, allowed the virus to continue to spread, create new variants, and harm others.

By mid-2021, after tens of millions of people had been vaccinated in the United States and billions around the world, it was clear that the new vaccines worked and were safe. Those who were hospitalized and died were invariably unvaccinated; states and counties with the highest vaccine rates had the lowest death rates. At this point in the pandemic, local health officials, colleges and universities, professional sports leagues, bars and restaurants, and many industries did the only thing they could have done to save lives: They mandated vaccines.

When someone steps on a rusty nail and pierces their foot, they are advised to get a tetanus shot. If they refuse, they are taking a risk—but the risk is personal. No one is going to catch tetanus from them; it's not a contagious disease. Covid is different. It *is* a contagious disease. Refusing to get a Covid vaccine is a choice to risk spreading the virus to others. Although vaccination doesn't eliminate the risk of transmitting the virus to others, it decreases that risk. People who refuse to get vaccinated are in essence saying, "It is my constitutional right to catch and transmit a potentially fatal infection." But is it?

ARE VACCINE MANDATES CONSTITUTIONAL?

In May 1899, a smallpox epidemic swept through the city of Boston, Massachusetts. By 1901, more than 200 Bostonians had fallen victim to the disease. In response, the Cambridge Board of Health proclaimed, "Whereas, smallpox has been prevalent in this city of Cambridge and has continued to increase; and whereas it is necessary for the speedy extermination of the disease; be it ordered that all inhabitants of the city be vaccinated." Citizens who refused were fined $5.00 (the equivalent of $175 today). In 1903, when the epidemic finally ended, smallpox had infected 1,600 people and killed 270. Had city health officials not acted quickly, the death toll would have been far greater.

One citizen, Henning Jacobson, a prominent Lutheran minister, refused to be vaccinated. Then he refused to pay the $5.00 fine. Jacobson's case worked its way up to the United States Supreme Court. The ruling in that case—called "the most important Supreme Court case in the history of American public health"—has been cited in more than 70 Supreme Court verdicts and, for more than a century, has determined whether states can force businesses to vaccinate their employees or parents to vaccinate their children.

On February 20, 1905, the Supreme Court—by a vote of 7 to 2—ruled that the right to refuse vaccination wasn't guaranteed by the Constitution. (The Constitution was written about 10 years *before* Edward Jenner created the world's first vaccine—the smallpox vaccine.) Representing the majority, Justice John Marshall Harlan argued that, in the arena of public health, societal good trumped individual freedoms: "The liberty secured by the Constitution of the United States to every person within its jurisdiction does not import an absolute right to each person to be ... wholly freed from restraint. There are manifold restraints to which every person is necessarily subject for the common good."

According to the U.S. Supreme Court, vaccine mandates were constitutional. In the realm of contagious diseases, public health was more important than individual freedoms. Indeed, during the Covid pandemic, many courts cited the 100-year-old ruling in *Jacobson* v. *Massachusetts* to uphold vaccine mandates.

CAN STATES LEGALLY MANDATE VACCINES FOR SCHOOL ENTRY?

Jacobson v. *Massachusetts* wasn't the last time that the Supreme Court considered the constitutionality of vaccine mandates. Seventeen years later, in 1922, officials from Brackenridge High School in San Antonio, Texas, expelled 15-year-old Rosalyn Zucht because her parents refused to give her the smallpox vaccine. Unlike Boston in the early 1900s, San Antonio wasn't suffering a smallpox epidemic; there was no public health emergency.

As it turned out, there didn't have to be. The mere threat of an outbreak was enough. In a unanimous decision, the Supreme Court reaffirmed the decision in *Jacobson* v. *Massachusetts,* ruling that Rosalyn's expulsion hadn't violated her constitutional rights. The decision in *Zucht* v. *King* reaffirmed the constitutionality of school vaccine mandates, which had been in place long before the *Jacobson* v. *Massachusetts* ruling.

Forty years passed.

In November 1966, public health officials determined that the time had come to eliminate measles from the United States. Their methods sparked a series of lawsuits.

Before the availability of a vaccine, measles infected millions of children in the United States every year and killed several hundred. But, with the invention of a measles vaccine in 1963, public health officials saw an opportunity. Because measles occurred primarily in school-aged children, health officials reasoned that the best way to eliminate it would be to mandate the vaccine for school entry. One prominent health official was photographed holding a sign that read, NO SHOTS, NO SCHOOL.

By the late 1960s, measles vaccination had caused a 95 percent drop in the incidence of the disease. By the early 1970s, however, immunization rates had become stagnant. Measles cases increased. In 1970, 47,000 cases were reported. By 1971, that figure had tripled. Although the number of states requiring vaccines for school entry increased from 25 in 1968 to 40 in 1974, health officials hadn't enforced those requirements. That would soon change:

- In 1976, during a massive measles outbreak in Alaska, state health officials informed parents that their children couldn't attend school until they were vaccinated. Fifty days later, when more than 7,400 students hadn't complied, school officials barred them from school. Within a month, fewer than 50 children remained unvaccinated and the epidemic ended.

• In 1977, during a measles outbreak in Los Angeles, thousands of children were infected. Many suffered measles pneumonia; three had measles encephalitis (inflammation of the brain), and two of those children died. On March 31, the county health director declared that any child who had not received a measles vaccine by May 2 would be excluded from school. When the deadline arrived, tens of thousands of students still hadn't been vaccinated. As had occurred the year before in Alaska, Los Angeles County parents soon realized that health officials weren't kidding—50,000 children were barred from school. Within days, most were back with proof of vaccination, again ending the epidemic.

• Perhaps the most dramatic example of the power of school mandates occurred in the twin cities of Texarkana, Texas, and Texarkana, Arkansas. Between June 1970 and January 1971, the Texarkana metropolitan areas suffered more than 600 cases of measles. Arkansas required vaccines for school entry; Texas didn't. Predictably, 96 percent of the cases occurred on the Texas side; 4 percent on the Arkansas side.

Vaccine mandates for school entry worked.

By 1981, all 50 states had school immunization requirements. By 2000, measles—one of the world's most contagious infectious diseases—was eliminated from the United States. But parents fought back against school mandates. As a result, measles has returned. By 2023, hundreds of people every year were again suffering from measles in the United States. The reason: A critical percentage of parents had chosen not to vaccinate their children.

How could this happen? Why did it happen?

Can Parents Legally Exempt Their Children From Vaccine Mandates?

School vaccine mandates provoked a backlash. Parents sued the states, claiming that their choice not to vaccinate their children was based on their religious beliefs. They argued that school mandates had violated their First Amendment rights, which guarantee that "Congress shall make no law respecting an establishment of religion, or prohibiting the free exercise thereof." The first few cases were unsuccessful.

Then an event occurred in Albany, New York, that opened a door.

Although it received scant media attention, on June 20, 1966, the New York State Assembly considered a bill requiring polio vaccine for school entry. The bill, which passed by a vote of 150 to 2, had an escape clause. It excluded children whose parents' religion forbade vaccination—a direct result of lobbying efforts by one of the most powerful religious groups in America: Christian Scientists. (The two legislators who voted against the bill, both Republicans, felt strongly that all children should be protected against polio, independent of the religious beliefs of their parents. Times have changed.)

The successful efforts by Christian Scientists to include a religious exemption in a New York State law changed the strategy of those who wanted to avoid vaccination. Plaintiffs now argued that it was unfair to allow vaccine exemptions for one religious group but not others. Religious exemptions were born. By 2009, 48 states had religious exemptions to vaccination.

Religious exemptions paved the way for another vaccine opt-out: philosophical exemptions. In the late 1980s, Louis Levy argued that the state should not be allowed to force his daughter, Sandra, to be vaccinated because vaccines were "a violation in a sense of our nature." The judge agreed, stating that vaccine exemptions could be granted if "beliefs [were] held with the strength of religious convictions," even if parents weren't members of a religious group. By 2009, 20 states had philosophical exemptions.

Only two states, Mississippi and West Virginia, didn't have religious or philosophical exemptions. Unless children in those two states had a medical exemption, they had to be vaccinated to attend private or public schools. As a result, Mississippi and West Virginia—states not known for their public health achievements—had the highest immunization rates in the country.

Then, starting in 2014, a measles outbreak in California caused the pendulum to swing in the other direction. For many Californians, the measles outbreak was the last straw. Five years earlier, the state had also suffered a whooping cough outbreak that killed 10 babies and sickened many others, all because parents had chosen not to vaccinate their children.

The California measles outbreak began when an unvaccinated boy developed measles following a December visit to the Disneyland Resort. By March, more than 130 people had been infected—virtually all in Southern California. The California outbreak spread to six other states, causing 16 more cases. Then the virus spread to Canada, causing 159 cases in a religious group in Québec. Another case linked to the California outbreak occurred in Mexico. The Disneyland case was also later linked to an ongoing measles outbreak in the Philippines.

In response to the California measles outbreak, a state senator and pediatrician named Richard Pan introduced Senate Bill 277, which eliminated California's personal belief exemption to vaccination. (California never had a religious exemption.) Despite vigorous protests from activists, Senate Bill 277 passed the California State Senate with a vote of 24 to 14. On June 30, 2015, Governor Jerry Brown signed it into law. California had become the third state, joining West Virginia and Mississippi, to allow only medical exemptions to vaccination. Connecticut, New York, and Maine soon followed. For parents living in those states who didn't want to vaccinate their children, the only option was homeschooling.

During committee hearings for Senate Bill 277, one seven-year-old boy became the voice of society. His name was Rhett Krawitt, and he was suffering from acute lymphoblastic leukemia. Standing on a chair so he could reach the microphone, Rhett explained that he was receiving chemotherapy, a medicine that eliminated his ability to respond to vaccines. "I depend on you to protect me," he said. "Don't I count?" Because they are immune compromised, about nine million people in the United States can't be vaccinated successfully. They depend on those around them to be vaccinated for protection.

SHOULD COVID VACCINES BE MANDATED POST-PANDEMIC?

Adults

When a Covid vaccine became widely available in early 2021, many industries were reluctant to mandate vaccines in the workplace. In a poll conducted in September 2021, 72 percent of those who were unvaccinated said that they would quit if forced to be vaccinated for work. News articles warned of mass resignations. Canadian truckers against vaccine mandates dominated the news cycle. Most businesses, fearing massive walk-offs, never mandated vaccines. These fears were understandable; by September 2021, more than 1,000 lawsuits opposing mandates had been filed against employers.

Reality, however, refuted those dire predictions. When large employers, school districts, and hospital systems finally mandated Covid vaccines, people got vaccinated, overwhelmingly. After United Airlines mandated Covid vaccines, only 200 holdouts occurred among its 67,000 employees. Among 10,000 employees in state-operated health care facilities in North Carolina, only 16 were fired for noncompliance.

By 2023, however, the situation in the United States had changed dramatically. In 2020, when SARS-CoV-2 first entered the United States, no one was immune; Americans were fully susceptible to this virus. Three years later, about 96 percent of the population was immune following Covid vaccination, natural infection, or both. No longer were 3,000 or 4,000 people dying every day. In response, restaurants, bars, and other businesses lifted vaccine requirements for their employees and patrons. So did most colleges and universities. By early 2023, at least 34 states had introduced bills that limited vaccine requirements.

If SARS-CoV-2 evolves to create a variant that is completely resistant to protection against severe disease afforded by previous infection or vaccination, vaccine mandates for the workplace might return. But until then, it is unlikely that adults employed outside of health care facilities will be required to receive a Covid vaccine.

One possible exception is the military. In December 2022, after Republicans had secured a majority in the House of Representatives, Kevin McCarthy, who would later become Speaker of the House, said that he would withhold annual funding to the military until it had removed Covid vaccine mandates. It will be the "first victory of the Republican Party," said McCarthy. In response, Defense Secretary Lloyd Austin countered, "We lost a million people to [SARS-CoV-2] virus. A million people died in the United States of America. We lost hundreds in [the Department of Defense]. So this mandate has kept people healthy."

The mandates caused problems, however. By early 2023, thousands of men had been refused entry to the military and more than 7,800 had been discharged because of their unwillingness to be vaccinated. Marine Corps general David Berger defended the vaccine mandate but worried that mandates were posing a problem for recruiting, especially in the South. On December 15, 2022, the United States Senate passed a bill rescinding Covid vaccine mandates for the military.

Although the crisis point of the pandemic had passed, for the winter semester of 2023, Harvard, Fordham, and the University of California schools, among others, still required a booster dose of a bivalent Covid vaccine to enter campus. Most universities didn't require booster dosing. Indeed, most hospitals didn't require booster dosing for employees.

The university booster requirements in the winter of 2023 didn't make much sense. If the goal of the vaccine was to prevent serious illness, healthy young people were unlikely to benefit as they didn't fall into a high-risk group. If the goal was to prevent mild illness for students living in dormitories, protection would likely last only a few months before antibodies faded.

Schoolchildren

In a post-pandemic world, Covid vaccine mandates in schools shouldn't be necessary. Knowing the following facts, all parents should want to vaccinate their young children:

1. Children can die from Covid; by April 2023, more than 1,700 children had succumbed to the disease.

2. Children between five and 13 years of age are those most likely to suffer from a post-infectious multisystem inflammatory syndrome (MIS-C) that causes severe heart, lung, liver, and kidney disease.

3. Children, like adults, can suffer from Covid for months (long Covid).

4. Covid vaccines, which have now been given to tens of millions of children, have been found to be highly effective at preventing severe illness and death.

5. Although Covid vaccines are a very rare cause of myocarditis, the problem appears to be short-lived and self-resolving. Myocarditis following Covid infection is more common and more severe than that following vaccination.

6. Between three and four million children are born every year in the United States who are fully susceptible to Covid by six months of age after immunity acquired from the mother through the placenta wanes.

7. SARS-CoV-2 is likely to circulate for decades.

8. Children are currently the least vaccinated group.

9. A study of more than 245,000 doses of Covid vaccine administered to children less than five years of age showed that the vaccine didn't cause any serious side effects, including myocarditis.

By the beginning of 2023, in the face of a receding pandemic, 96 percent population immunity, and markedly reduced numbers of hospitalizations and deaths, only a few schools for young children in California and the District of Columbia still had vaccine mandates. Like mandates for adults in the workplace, unless a variant emerges that completely evades protection against severe disease afforded by vaccination or previous infection, school mandates are unlikely to return.

One series of events, however, has been particularly worrisome.

As the pandemic was subsiding, comments from Republican legislators and right-wing media pundits revealed an interest in ending not only Covid vaccine mandates for children, but also all school vaccine mandates. It started with comments made by Big Bird.

In early November 2021, after the CDC had approved vaccines for five- to 11-year-olds, the *Sesame Street* character Big Bird tweeted, "I got the Covid-19 vaccine today! My wing is feeling a little sore, but it'll give my body an extra protective boost that keeps me and others healthy."

A few days later, Big Bird found himself the victim of an attack by Ted Cruz, a Republican senator from Texas, who tweeted, "Government propaganda ... for your 5-year-old!" Cruz said that although "I support the vaccine and have received it," he opposed mandates imposed by President Biden and that schools should not be involved in vaccinating kids. (U.S. presidents can't mandate vaccines; mandates can only occur at the state and local level.) Following Ted Cruz's lead, Wendy Rogers, a Republican state senator from Arizona, tweeted, "Big Bird is a communist." (Begging the question, what does she say about Mr. Snuffleupagus?)

Since 1969, Big Bird—the beloved eight-foot-tall anthropomorphic yellow bird who is perpetually six and a half years old—has helped generations of children build self-confidence, confront fear, and deal with loss (after the death of Mr. Hooper). Not surprisingly, he has never been at the center of a political controversy.

What had Big Bird done to incur the wrath of these legislators? He certainly wasn't the first celebrity to encourage children to be vaccinated. Nor was he the most famous. On October 28, 1956, before taking the stage on the *Ed Sullivan Show* to play "Hound Dog," Elvis Presley received a polio vaccine on national television. The Presley appearance was designed to convince teenagers to get vaccinated. It worked. By August 1957, about 75 percent of Americans under 20 had received the vaccine.

Celebrity endorsements continued. In 1977, the *Star Wars* characters C-3PO and R2-D2 were part of a public health campaign. "Immunize your children, please," said C-3PO, "and may the Force be with you." In the 1980s, the popular author of children's books, Roald Dahl, advocated for childhood vaccines after the death of his daughter from measles. Today, celebrities such as Seth MacFarlane, Amanda Peet, Dolly Parton, Joan Collins, Samuel L. Jackson, Willie Nelson, Tyler Perry, and Mariah Carey have all actively supported vaccines for children. Indeed, Big Bird's promotion of Covid vaccines wasn't his first. In 1972, he read a sign on *Sesame Street* that stated, "Don't wait. Vaccinate."

So, why did Ted Cruz and Wendy Rogers attack Big Bird? The answer can be found in a celebrity endorsement in 1978, when school vaccine mandates were first being put in place across the country. "Get your kids shots," said legendary boxer Muhammad Ali. "The law says if your kids don't have their shots for dangerous diseases like measles, mumps, and polio, they aren't getting into school. The law also says they must go to school. So, you have no choice. Get your kids their shots."

Ali had touched the third rail of what has energized and galvanized the political Right: freedom of choice. Nothing incites stronger, angrier, more volatile feelings among the Right than the perception of government control.

On October 20, 2022, after the CDC's vaccine advisory committee recommended that Covid vaccines be added to the childhood immunization schedule, Tucker Carlson joined the fray, tweeting, "The CDC is about to add the Covid vaccine to the childhood immunization schedule, which would make the vax mandatory for kids to attend school."

Carlson was right that the CDC would likely follow the advisory committee's advice and recommend the Covid vaccine for children. But he was wrong to claim that the CDC had the power to mandate vaccines for school entry. The CDC quickly refuted Carlson's claim, tweeting, "States require vaccines for school children, not the CDC." In other words, the decision of whether to mandate Covid vaccines is up to the states; there are no federal vaccine mandates for children. For example, although the CDC also recommends the influenza vaccine for all children more than six months of age, no state requires the vaccine for school entry. Covid vaccines may well fall into that category.

During 2022, fueled by the political Right, state and local legislatures had introduced more bills opposing vaccine mandates for school entry than ever before. If these challenges to school vaccine mandates are successful, we will likely return to a time when highly contagious diseases once again cause thousands of hospitalizations and hundreds of deaths.

As an example, in July 2022, a 27-year-old unvaccinated man living in an Orthodox Jewish community in Rockland County, New York—which had immunization rates of around 30 percent—was paralyzed by polio. Only 1 of every 2,000 people infected with the type of poliovirus that had infected this man will be paralyzed; the rest will have an asymptomatic, mild, or short-lived illness. Therefore, this case of paralysis represented the tip of a much larger iceberg of polio infections. Indeed, poliovirus was detected in Rockland County wastewater as well as in the wastewater of several surrounding counties.

In 2019, activists filed 221 bills relating to vaccines in state legislatures across the country; in 2020, 232; in 2021, 473; and in 2022, 875, more than in any previous year in U.S. history. More than half the bills filed in 2022 opposed mandates for all vaccines. By December 2022, more than a third of parents believed that school vaccine mandates should be eliminated.

It's a dangerous game to play, and a game we're already playing.

CHAPTER 13

....

IS IMMUNITY FROM NATURAL INFECTION BETTER THAN VACCINATION?

- Is immunity after any natural infection better than vaccination?
- Is immunity after a natural Covid infection better than a Covid vaccine?
- Was it reasonable to have mandated Covid vaccines for people who had been naturally infected?

When Robert Malone appeared on Joe Rogan's podcast, the following exchange occurred:

> **Rogan:** *So, if they had just done what Sweden had done and some other countries where they didn't institute lockdowns and they sort of let people just live their lives and make their own choices, they were saying that millions of people wouldn't have died?*
>
> **Malone:** *So it would be. So, it seems.*
>
> **Rogan:** *But time has shown that Sweden actually had a more effective take on the virus.*

Throughout this chapter, I will use the term "natural immunity" to refer to immunity induced by infection, although I do so reluctantly. Millions of people have died from Covid. So, I think the better term would be "survivor immunity," or at least "infection-induced immunity."

The word "natural" has a nice sound. Many products are sold with phrases like "all natural." But nothing good comes from being infected with viruses that could send you to the hospital, intensive care unit, or morgue or can cause lifelong disabilities. Polio is natural. So are smallpox and malaria. Indeed, Mother Nature has been trying to kill us ever since we crawled out of the ocean onto land. (I would really like to know the name of Mother Nature's public relations firm, because they're doing a great job.)

At the beginning of the pandemic, Swedish health officials isolated only those who were at highest risk of severe Covid, arguing that natural infection would be the best way to encourage population immunity and slow the spread of the virus. Sweden was probably right not to close schools for young children, who were at the lowest risk of severe disease. Indeed, in the United States, children denied school entry early in the pandemic suffered mightily from a lack of education and socialization. Some parents argued reasonably that the cure might have been worse than the disease.

But Robert Malone and Joe Rogan shouldn't have been so quick to praise Swedish health officials. Compared with other countries in Europe, Sweden's death rates were a little better than the middle of the pack. Compared with other Scandinavian countries, however, Sweden was one of the worst, with death rates about 10 times higher than those of neighboring Norway and twice as high as those in Denmark. Nursing home residents and immigrants in Sweden were particularly vulnerable. In 2022, researchers at the Karolinska Institute, which awards the Nobel Prizes, argued that public health officials in Sweden should be held accountable for their failures.

Early in the pandemic, Sweden wasn't the only country interested in removing public health restraints and letting natural infections take their course. In August 2020, Donald Trump selected Dr. Scott Atlas, a radiologist and senior fellow in health policy at Stanford University's Hoover Institution, to serve as an adviser to the White House's Coronavirus Task Force. Among his many controversial statements, Atlas, like Swedish health officials, argued that population (or herd) immunity was best achieved by allowing the virus to spread among groups least likely to die from the disease. He argued that only about 20 percent of the population would need to be naturally infected to slow the spread of the virus. Atlas's estimate was low. Really low. As it turned out, about 95 percent of the population had to be immune to dramatically reduce the number of hospitalizations and deaths from Covid.

In January 2022, Anthony Fauci wondered aloud whether the Omicron variant, which appeared to be highly contagious but less lethal, was "the live viral vaccine we have all been hoping for"—again, arguing that immunity from natural infection might be the most efficient way to achieve better, longer-lasting protection. As it turned out, a study in Hong Kong published in June 2023 showed that the hospitalization rates in people who had not been vaccinated or naturally infected were the same during the Alpha, Delta, and Omicron waves. Omicron wasn't less lethal.

IS IMMUNITY AFTER ANY NATURAL INFECTION BETTER THAN VACCINATION?

As a child of the 1950s, I had measles, as did millions of children my age every year. My children, on the other hand, who were born in the 1990s, never had measles; instead, they received two doses of the measles vaccine. The quantity of my memory immune cells following natural infection is probably greater than that of my vaccinated children. In other words, I probably have better immunity against measles than my children.

The goal of all vaccines is to induce the immunity that follows natural infection *without paying the price of natural infection*. Though I paid the price, I was lucky. I wasn't one of the 48,000 people who were hospitalized and 500 who died every year from measles in the United States.

So, the question isn't, "Is immunity after natural measles infection better than vaccination?" It generally is. The better question is, "Is immunity after measles vaccination good enough?" The answer to the second question is clearly yes. Because of the measles vaccine, measles was eliminated from the United States by 2000. No longer did children have to pay such a high price for immunity. No longer did they have to suffer and die every year from the virus. Because measles virus has a long incubation period (see chapter 8), both my children and I will likely be protected against all symptomatic measles infections, even mild infections, for the rest of our lives.

Unfortunately, because a critical percentage of parents are now choosing not to vaccinate their children, measles has crept back. At the end of December 2022, schools and day care centers in Columbus, Ohio, reported 85 cases of measles in children, 70 percent of which occurred in those less than two years of age. Thirty-two children were hospitalized; all were unvaccinated. As is so often the case, the most vulnerable among us suffer our ignorance.

Several years ago, I spoke at a conference in Jacksonville, Florida. During the question-and-answer session, one anti-vaccine activist in the audience said, "I had measles and I'm fine. And so are many of the people in this room." He then gestured to those sitting around him.

Unfortunately, those who could have best countered his argument weren't in the audience. Not as lucky as this man, they weren't alive to tell their stories. Put another way, natural immunity is valuable so long as you don't die acquiring it. Many people in car accidents walk away unscathed. This doesn't mean that car accidents aren't dangerous; it only means that some people are lucky.

IS IMMUNITY AFTER A NATURAL COVID INFECTION BETTER THAN A COVID VACCINE?

Covid vaccines induce antibodies, as well as memory B and T cells, directed against the SARS-CoV-2 spike protein. People who are naturally infected also develop antibodies and memory B and T cells against the spike protein, as well as the other three SARS-CoV-2 proteins. Therefore, it would stand to reason that people who were naturally infected, like those who were vaccinated, would be protected against mild disease for a few months and severe disease for years.

Between 2021 and 2022, when the Alpha, Delta, and Omicron variants were circulating in the United States, more than a dozen studies showed that natural infection and vaccination were both highly effective at preventing severe Covid. Probably the best study, which was published by Harvard University researchers in *Science Immunology* on May 12, 2022, showed that the broadest, longest-lasting, protective immune response to Covid was induced by either three doses of an mRNA vaccine or two doses of an mRNA vaccine plus a natural infection.

WAS IT REASONABLE TO HAVE MANDATED COVID VACCINES FOR PEOPLE WHO HAD BEEN NATURALLY INFECTED?

People who had been naturally infected with Covid during the time when mandates were enforced argued that they were protected against the disease. They reasoned that proof of immunity to hepatitis B virus was good enough for hospitals that required the hepatitis B vaccine for employment; the same was true for hospitals that required measles and chicken pox vaccines. So, why not allow proof of immunity following SARS-CoV-2 infection as an opt-out for mandated Covid vaccination?

On February 2, 2022, public health officials from the CDC, NIH, and the Biden administration held a meeting with a handful of immunologists, virologists, and vaccine experts to determine whether proof of natural infection should count as a vaccination. This was a highly contentious issue. Some people who had been naturally infected were denied access to public venues or were losing their jobs because they had refused to be vaccinated.

Imagine that you were part of this meeting. As a participant, you would have been asked to weigh the following facts:

- During the week that the meeting took place, 2,500 Americans had died from Covid.

- A study in Kentucky had shown that vaccination boosted and extended immunity to Covid in those who had been previously infected.

- Proof of natural infection could be provided either by showing a positive PCR or antigen test, or by showing evidence of antibodies in the blood directed against the SARS-CoV-2 nucleoprotein, all of which could be easily faked or purchased off the internet.

- Many venues, like hospitals, nursing homes, and chronic care facilities, mandated vaccines because they were responsible for those at highest risk of serious disease. If caregivers faked a previous infection, those in their care were particularly vulnerable.

• Providing proof of immunity was yet another administrative hurdle at a time when existing bureaucracy already overwhelmed many.

The session ended with a split decision. Some were in favor of allowing natural infection to count (I was one of those people); others weren't. In retrospect, it would have been reasonable not to mandate vaccination for people who had been previously infected, especially considering they might be barred from work for refusing vaccination. But hindsight is always 20/20. And those who argued against natural infection as an opt-out pointed to the fact that vaccinating those who had already been infected would only enhance and broaden immunity.

CHAPTER 14
••••••••••••••

A PRACTICAL GUIDE TO COVID TODAY

- Can we stop testing and masking?
- Who should receive Covid vaccines and boosters?
- Should Covid vaccines be tailored to the circulating strains?
- Should Covid vaccines be offered every year, like influenza vaccines?

This book was completed in June 2023. The advice that follows is based on the following assumptions:

1. SARS-CoV-2 continues to circulate the world.

2. SARS-CoV-2 continues to create variants. However, none of these variants resists protection against severe disease following immunization or natural infection in otherwise healthy people.

3. SARS-CoV-2 variants might become less virulent but not avirulent, meaning that people infected with these new strains could still be hospitalized and die. In other words, SARS-CoV-2 doesn't become another common cold virus.

4. The number of people hospitalized or killed by Covid every year begins to resemble that of influenza, respiratory syncytial virus (RSV), and the other winter respiratory viruses.

5. Virtually everyone in the United States continues to act as they did before the pandemic, no longer changing the way they live, work, or play. Schools and businesses remain open. Large outdoor and indoor sporting events occur without restrictions.

Assuming all these things are true, how can we continue to protect those who are most susceptible to dying from Covid? Specifically, how can we protect the 54 million Americans who are over 75; the 1.2 million living in nursing homes; the millions with high-risk medical conditions such as chronic lung, heart, or kidney disease; the nine million who are severely immune compromised and don't adequately respond to Covid vaccines; and the three to four million babies born every year who, by six months of age, will be fully susceptible to this virus?

CAN WE STOP TESTING AND MASKING?

Every winter, viruses such as influenza, respiratory syncytial virus (RSV), human metapneumovirus, parainfluenza virus, adenovirus, human coronaviruses, rhinovirus, and others cause tens of thousands of people to suffer, be hospitalized, and die. The only year that this didn't occur was 2020. By closing businesses, shuttering schools, isolating, quarantining, masking, and restricting travel, we essentially eliminated many of these winter respiratory viruses, which tells you how much worse Covid might have been had we not implemented those restrictions. In the winter of 2022–23, respiratory viruses returned—some, with a vengeance. RSV overwhelmed many pediatric and adult hospitals and intensive care units, as did influenza.

What should we do now for people who have congestion, cough, sore throat, runny nose, fever, muscle aches, and joint aches—all symptoms of Covid, as well as these other winter viruses? As of 2023, the CDC recommended that people with respiratory symptoms test for Covid and, if positive, isolate themselves until they are symptom free and testing negative. The CDC also suggested that people who are exposed to someone known to have Covid or are about to encounter someone at high risk of severe Covid should test themselves.

Should we continue with these recommendations indefinitely? Frankly, even if these CDC recommendations remained in place through 2024 and beyond, few would follow them.

Here's another way of approaching this. If you have symptoms of a respiratory viral infection, and are in a high-risk group, test for Covid. If you have Covid, take an antiviral medicine early in the illness. If you aren't in a high-risk group, don't test for Covid.

During the pandemic, many people felt that if they had respiratory symptoms but tested negative for Covid, they could go about their daily activities as before, comfortable that they weren't spreading a harmful virus. This didn't make much sense. Other winter respiratory viruses can be similarly deadly. For example, every year in the United States:

- Influenza causes 140,000 to 800,000 hospitalizations and 12,000 to 60,000 deaths—100 to 200 of those deaths occur in children.

- RSV causes about 80,000 hospitalizations in children and 100 to 300 deaths. In the elderly, RSV causes between

100,000 and 180,000 hospitalizations and 8,000 and 14,000 deaths.

- Parainfluenza virus causes about 70,000 hospitalizations and 440 deaths.

In other words, you don't have to be infected with Covid to be sick or die or transmit a virus that could harm or kill others.

As Covid hospitalization and death rates are now approaching the rates of these other viruses, wouldn't it make sense to treat them all the same? Given this, I recommend that if you have symptoms consistent with a viral respiratory tract infection, such as sore throat, congestion, cough, or fever (and aren't in a high-risk group), just assume that you have Covid or one of these other respiratory viruses and stay home until you no longer have significant symptoms, especially fever. If you can't stay home, wear a mask until your symptoms are gone, and have children who can wear a mask do the same. Masks clearly decrease transmission of the virus; they aren't fool-proof, but they are much better than not masking. For those who can't or won't wear a mask, keep them home until they are significantly better.

This is the best way to lessen the burden of these terrible diseases. This approach would mean a dramatic change from what we have been doing. But it makes more sense than treating Covid differently from these other infections when all can be harmful. Also, given that transmission of virus can occur *before* symptoms develop, prevention of transmission won't be absolute.

At some point in the future, a rapid home test might be available for all respiratory viruses. Then those in high-risk groups can know whether they should treat themselves for Covid (with Paxlovid or remdesivir) or influenza (with Tamiflu).

WHO SHOULD RECEIVE
COVID VACCINES AND BOOSTERS?

Vaccines

Because SARS-CoV-2 and its many variants will continue to circulate the world for decades, if not longer, everyone more than six months of age is at risk of severe illness and should be vaccinated. For people who have been naturally infected but never vaccinated, two doses of an mRNA-containing vaccine will broaden and lengthen immunity. For people who have never been naturally infected, three doses of a Covid vaccine are as effective as two doses plus a natural infection (see chapter 13). These recommendations might change as different vaccines become available.

Pregnant people represent a special group of adults who should be vaccinated during every pregnancy. First, to protect themselves. Pregnant people are much more likely to be hospitalized, admitted to the intensive care unit, placed on a ventilator, and die from Covid than people of the same age who aren't pregnant. Second, although the CDC now recommends Covid vaccines for children, these vaccines aren't available for babies younger than six months of age. People who receive a Covid vaccine during pregnancy will develop protective antibodies in their bloodstream that, beginning at around 32 weeks gestation, will be passively transferred to their baby through the placenta. These antibodies will protect babies in the first six months of life, before they are able to receive a vaccine. During the fall of 2022, babies were the group of children most likely to be hospitalized with Covid, primarily with croup and bronchiolitis (inflammation of the small breathing tubes in the lungs).

Pregnant people reasonably worry whether the vaccine given during pregnancy will be safe for their baby. But studies have shown the mRNA vaccines, which are contained in lipid nanoparticles, don't enter the baby's bloodstream. Also, millions of people have now been vaccinated during pregnancy. Tens of thousands of these people have been compared with pregnant individuals who didn't receive the vaccine to determine differences in pregnancy outcomes (such as miscarriages) or neonatal outcomes (such as birth defects). No differences were found. The only difference was that pregnant people who were vaccinated were less likely to suffer severe Covid and more likely to have babies who were protected against the disease.

Boosters

The question of who should receive Covid boosters depends on how long protection against severe disease lasts. Four groups appeared to benefit from booster vaccines given in the fall and winter of 2022–23: people who were immune compromised, people who had high-risk medical conditions, people older than 75, and pregnant people. Booster doses of a vaccine lessened the risk that people in these groups would be hospitalized or killed by Covid. These groups will likely continue to benefit from a Covid vaccine given every fall. But it remains incumbent upon the CDC and academic researchers to prove that.

How about everyone else? Should healthy people less than 75 years of age who have received three doses of vaccine or two doses plus a natural infection also receive a yearly vaccine to lessen their risk of hospitalization? By the middle of 2023, the answer to that question was no, but that might change. It is again up to the CDC to determine how long protective immunity against severe disease lasts for younger, healthy people. These CDC studies should be done in concert with academic immunologists who can, at the same time, determine how long memory B and T cells last. These are the immune cells that likely best correlate with protection against severe disease.

Researchers must also determine how long protection against severe disease lasts for children who were vaccinated between six months and five years of age. Or between five years and 11 years of age. Or between 11 years and 17 years of age. Are all groups the same? Does the age of vaccination determine how long immunity lasts? Also, how long does protection against severe disease last for people who have been vaccinated but not naturally infected, or naturally infected but not vaccinated, or both vaccinated and naturally infected?

Moving forward, we need to understand these issues. We shouldn't vaccinate everyone every year just because we don't know. In the years ahead, it is incumbent upon the CDC to determine who is being hospitalized and killed by Covid. What are their ages? What is their immunization status? At what age were they first vaccinated? How long ago were they boosted? Did they have other medical problems? Did they take antiviral medicines? Only with this knowledge will we learn who needs to receive booster dosing and who doesn't.

I'm under 75 and otherwise healthy. I have received three doses of a Covid vaccine; the last dose was given in November 2021. Six months later, in May 2022, I had a mild Covid illness caused by one of the Omicron variants (probably BA.2). I will likely be protected against severe Covid for years. But I don't know that. And I need to know. I will look to the CDC and academic researchers to determine how long immunity against severe disease lasts for people like me and then, and only then, will I get a booster dose.

SHOULD COVID VACCINES BE TAILORED TO THE CIRCULATING STRAINS?

By the beginning of 2023, there was little reason to include Wuhan-1 (the ancestral strain) in Covid vaccines. Covid vaccines will likely be tailored to the circulating strain or strains in either monovalent, bivalent, or multivalent vaccines. The advantage of moving away from the ancestral strain in vaccines is that the ancestral strain is gone and unlikely to return. Also, for people who have never been vaccinated or naturally infected, vaccinating with strains that are circulating will provide much better protection against mild illness, at least in the short term. Tailoring the vaccines to the circulating strains would also be of value to those who are so medically frail that even a mild infection could land them in the hospital.

In May 2023, the WHO recommended that Covid vaccines contain only one of the Omicron strains. In June 2023, the FDA's vaccine advisory committee recommended that the 2023–24 Covid vaccine contain one of the Omicron variants (XBB.1.5) and that the vaccine would no longer contain the original ancestral strain.

SHOULD COVID VACCINES BE OFFERED EVERY YEAR, LIKE INFLUENZA VACCINES?

Every year, the CDC recommends an influenza vaccine for anyone over six months of age. That's because influenza viruses change so much from one year to the next that natural infection or immunization the year before doesn't protect against severe disease. Like Covid vaccines, the goal of influenza vaccines is to keep people out of the hospital, out of the intensive care unit, and out of the morgue.

To determine which strains to include in the yearly influenza vaccine, members of the FDA's vaccine advisory committee gather in the first week of March to listen to presentations by the Department of Defense, WHO, FDA, and CDC. Presentations focus on which influenza strains are circulating in countries in the Southern Hemisphere, such as Australia and South America, where winters precede those in the United States. Influenza strains circulating in these countries around March often predict which strains the

United States will see in September. After the decision is made on which strains to include, companies make the vaccine—a process that takes about six months. If the FDA advisory committee incorrectly predicts which strains to include in the annual influenza vaccine, which has happened three times in the past 20 years, the results can be disastrous; a miss is a mile. Vaccine efficacy against severe influenza when the strains in the vaccine didn't match the circulating strains was less than 15 percent. In other words, protection against severe influenza is strain-specific.

Is SARS-CoV-2 similar enough to influenza virus to require a yearly vaccine? Asked another way, does SARS-CoV-2 change so much from one year to the next that people who were previously vaccinated or naturally infected or both are no longer protected against severe illness? At the beginning of 2023, the answer was no. Healthy young people who had been vaccinated against SARS-CoV-2 remained protected against severe disease the following year because, although new variants continued to evolve, the parts of the virus that were recognized by T cells remained virtually unchanged (see chapter 8). Unlike influenza, protection against serious disease has not, thus far, been strain-specific.

LESSONS LEARNED (OR NOT)

Will our experiences with SARS-CoV-2, which by the beginning of 2023 had killed a little less than seven million people worldwide, prepare us better for the next pandemic? The following lists some of the painful lessons—and a few wins—from the Covid experience.

LESSON #1: SURVEILLANCE

Although some continue to debate whether SARS-CoV-2 was a product of nature or a product of man (which at this point is no longer debatable), one thing is clear—the virus originated in China. And China waited far too long to tell the world that a novel virus was killing thousands of people. We need a robust international surveillance system that doesn't depend on one nation acting responsibly. This system could be directed by scientists and public health officials representing all countries and regions of the world. China's reluctance to allow scientists from other countries to examine what was happening in Wuhan only fueled conspiracy theories and further delayed our understanding of this virus.

LESSON #2: GETTING READY FOR THE ONSLAUGHT

The United States is a technologically advanced, wealthy country. Early in the pandemic, however, it didn't act like one. Nurses were wearing bandannas and plastic bags when proper face masks and gowns were unavailable. States were fighting with each other to procure ventilators. Hospitals were overwhelmed. Accurate and reliable Covid test kits were delayed.

Once it had become clear that a pandemic was at hand, President Trump should have immediately used his authority through the Defense Production Act to order the manufacture of masks, gowns, and ventilators and to provide resources to create more hospital space. Also, instead of making its own test kits, which took far too long and were initially inaccurate, the CDC should have enlisted the help of commercial laboratories. These problems were easily solved. Several other countries did a far better job of preparing for and responding to the Covid pandemic than the United States.

LESSON #3: OPERATION WARP SPEED

Perhaps the brightest point of light during the Covid pandemic was Operation Warp Speed. Only 11 months after SARS-CoV-2 was isolated, two vaccines had been tested in large clinical trials and found to be safe and effective. Later, the White House successfully partnered with pharmacies and hospitals to distribute and administer vaccines, as well as provide test kits and antivirals. It was an amazing effort and bodes well for our ability to create and distribute vaccines against future pandemic viruses.

LESSON #4: VACCINATING THE WORLD

The United States has the technological capacity and resources to vaccinate the world. It wouldn't be an altruistic act. SARS-CoV-2 will continue to circulate and continue to create variants for decades to come. Indeed, at the beginning of 2023, more than one-third of the people living on the planet had not received a single dose of a Covid vaccine. The degree to which other countries are at risk for severe disease is the degree to which we are all at risk. No one is safe until everyone is safe.

LESSON #5: GETTING THE PUBLIC TO UNDERSTAND THE SCIENTIFIC PROCESS

When I was a pediatric resident at the Children's Hospital of Philadelphia, I learned that babies should be placed on their stomachs after eating. That way, if they regurgitated breast milk or infant formula, they wouldn't aspirate it into their lungs. Bad advice. As it turned out, babies were more likely to die of sudden infant death syndrome (SIDS) if they slept on their stomachs than on their backs.

In the early 1990s, about 10 years after I finished my pediatric residency—when it had become clear that babies were more likely to die from SIDS if they slept on their stomachs—the American Academy of Pediatrics launched its "Back to Sleep" campaign, encouraging parents to place babies on their back to sleep. The incidence of SIDS plummeted. What I had learned during my pediatric residency was wrong. This didn't mean that the senior physicians who taught me pediatrics were bad doctors. It only meant that we learn as we go. As is true for every aspect of science and medicine.

Recommendations for the treatment and prevention of Covid have evolved as we've learned more about how SARS-CoV-2 is transmitted and who is at greatest risk. For example, early in the pandemic it was unclear exactly how the virus was spread. Was it spread solely by small droplets from the nose and mouth? Or could the virus also live on surfaces, like cans in a grocery store? We were told to wash our hands constantly and clean surfaces and store-bought items. Eventually, it became clear that while masking was important, washing and cleaning had a lesser impact.

Scientists, clinicians, and public health officials should be careful to inform the public that all recommendations are based on what we know at the time and that things might change. Otherwise, the fluidity of scientific knowledge will remain disconcerting. We learn as we go. This will always be true.

LESSON #6: STOP THE SPREAD OF MISINFORMATION

Good luck with this one. It's like trying to stop the devastation of Hurricane Katrina with a plastic cup. If social media continue to provide a platform for misinformation, which is inevitable, this will remain an impossible task. The good news is that many websites, blogs, webinars, videos, and podcasts provide excellent counters to misinformation for people looking to fact-check. We should do everything possible to keep these responsible sites front and center.

LESSON #7: GRASS ROOTS
CAMPAIGNS CAN ENGENDER TRUST

Although countering misinformation at a national or statewide level is virtually impossible, it's possible at a local level. During the Covid pandemic, Dr. Ala Stanford showed us the way. She and her Black Doctors Covid-19 Consortium (BDCC) sat in people's homes in North Philadelphia and provided residents with a consistent and trustworthy source of information. And, in a community resistant to vaccination, she and her colleagues reassured and educated more than 50,000 residents to vaccinate themselves and their children. It's one of the many heartening moments during this pandemic.

LESSON #8: SEPARATE POLITICS AND SCIENCE

Again, good luck with this one.

For the first time in human history, deaths from a vaccine-preventable disease were divided along party lines. As of December 2022, 37 percent of Republicans but only 9 percent of Democrats were unvaccinated. Seventeen of the 18 states with the lowest vaccine rates voted for Donald Trump in 2020; not surprisingly, these were the states that had the highest death rates from Covid per capita. Republicans in positions of power who discouraged vaccination were complicit in the premature deaths of their followers. (Because it's about resources and values, public health will always to some extent be political. But it doesn't have to be partisan.)

If, as is currently the case, politicians believe they can garner more votes by sounding a libertarian, government-off-my-back, ignore-public-health-officials, vaccines-are-dangerous, no-vaccine-mandates diatribe, they'll do it. Politicians are rarely statesmen; rather, they're the wetted-finger-to-the-wind crowd, perfectly willing to tell their constituents what they want to hear, even if it puts everyone's health at risk. Or, as historian John Barry notes, "When you mix politics with science, you get politics."

Trying to get politicians to act like statesmen, instead of shilling for the biggest applause lines, will be about as easy as teaching algebra to goldfish.

LESSON #9: FOLLOW THE SCIENCE

Donald Trump's arm twisting to approve hydroxychloroquine was a sad day for FDA officials, whose job is to protect the American public from products that are unsafe or ineffective—which, in the case of hydroxychloroquine, was both. And Trump's promotion of bleach as a cure for Covid was a grotesque parody of the scientific process.

In the wake of these disastrous decisions, the Biden administration promised to "follow the science." But in several instances, his administration also made mistakes. The use of the term "breakthrough" to describe a mild or asymptomatic infection set an unrealistic bar for Covid vaccines. Similarly, the continued promotion of the bivalent vaccine booster in 2022 as better than the monovalent vaccine wasn't supported by evidence.

Many in the academic community stood up to question the administration's message, pointing to the science. As a result, the public was confused. At this point, the administration should have admitted its mistakes. It's OK to be wrong. And it's OK to change recommendations when new data are available. But don't keep doubling down, which only further erodes trust—not only from the public, but also from members of the scientific and medical community.

It's not hard to fix this. Public health officials need to quickly update recommendations based on new data, no matter how painful or contradictory to what was previously believed to be true. Educate about the reasoning behind the change, and then trust the American public to understand that some recommendations might change when dealing with viruses or vaccines with which we've had little previous experience.

None of the mistakes the Trump and Biden administrations made were nefarious. President Trump believed that hydroxychloroquine was a lifesaver, and President Biden believed that a bivalent vaccine containing the circulating strains was better than what we had. The bivalent vaccines in 2022–23 were certainly as good as the monovalent vaccines. And they were important in keeping those at highest risk out of the hospital. Moving forward, Covid vaccines will likely be constructed in a manner that clearly makes them better. But in the meantime, public health officials don't need to overstate claims of efficacy.

LESSON #10: PRIORITIZE THE MOST VULNERABLE

Although everyone at every age is susceptible to Covid, not everyone is equally susceptible to serious illness. Elderly adults suffered a death rate about a thousandfold greater than children; indeed, about 40 percent of all Covid deaths occurred in nursing homes. Similarly, studies of booster dosing showed that those most likely to benefit included people over 75, people with multiple health problems, people who were immune compromised, and pregnant people. For as long as this virus circulates, the primary focus should be on protecting these four groups.

LESSON #11: DON'T IGNORE
THE POWER OF ANTIVIRALS

One problem with the groups at highest risk of dying from Covid is that many don't develop a good immune response to vaccination—no matter how many times they are boosted. For that reason, when the focus was almost solely on boosting and boosting and boosting those high-risk groups, antivirals were underemphasized. Consequently, many deaths were avoidable. False notions about the harms caused by Paxlovid also limited uptake. Indeed, so prevalent was the fear of Paxlovid that in November 2022, *The Atlantic* wrote a piece titled, "Inside the Mind of an Anti-Paxxer." Unlike anti-vaccine activists, anti-Paxxers were not aligned with the political Right. Rather, the single driving force against using Paxlovid was fear of Paxlovid rebound, which isn't a real thing.

LESSON #12: THE CURE SHOULDN'T
BE WORSE THAN THE DISEASE

Early in the pandemic, when antivirals, monoclonal antibodies, and vaccines weren't available, the only strategy for decreasing Covid was limiting human-to-human contact. We closed businesses and shuttered schools. No one paid a bigger price for this strategy than children, who suffered severely from the lack of education and socialization; the impact of these deficits will no doubt be felt for years to come. Our interest in getting children back to school should have been just as intense as our interest in getting people back to work. Indeed, early in the pandemic, the American Academy of Pediatrics recommended against school closures, which as it turned out, was probably the best advice.

LESSON #13: DON'T BYPASS
VACCINE ADVISORY COMMITTEES

During the pandemic, the production and testing of vaccines were performed quickly. Occasionally, independent vaccine advisory committees like the CDC's Advisory Committee on Immunization Practices (ACIP) or the FDA's vaccine advisory committee were bypassed—especially regarding recommendations about booster dosing and bivalent vaccines.

This is never a good idea. The advantage of seeking advice from these committees, in addition to the fact that they are composed of scientists and clinicians who are independent of both the government and pharmaceutical companies, is that committee hearings are open to the public. Anyone can watch the deliberations online. This allows everyone, including the media, to hear discussions about the strengths and weaknesses of the science behind specific policy decisions. Also, all the materials presented at these meetings are available to the public.

LESSON #14: IMPROVE CDC SURVEILLANCE SYSTEMS

Throughout the pandemic, we needed to know much more about who was being hospitalized and who was dying from Covid. What were their ages, ethnic backgrounds, vaccination status, booster status, and underlying health problems? Had they received antivirals or monoclonal antibodies? Where did they live?

Wastewater analysis would have given us a heads-up on potential Covid surges, as well as the variants that would likely be associated with those surges. This kind of information was critical for making decisions about vaccines and antivirals, but it was slow in coming. Indeed, public health officials often relied on data generated in Canada, Israel, and the United Kingdom, all of which had national health systems.

During the pandemic, it became clear that some patients said to be admitted for Covid weren't admitted because they had Covid. Rather, they were admitted for other reasons and just happened to be infected, often asymptomatically, at the same time. A study performed in Massachusetts, Pennsylvania, and Illinois, in which all hospital admissions for Covid were thoroughly reviewed, found that at least 25 percent of what had been counted as Covid hospitalizations were incidental infections. In some instances, rates of incidental Covid were as high as 75 percent.

In December 2022, to obtain more reliable information as to who was and wasn't hospitalized for Covid, a prestigious infectious diseases group called the Society for Healthcare Epidemiology of America requested that all hospitals discontinue routine Covid testing on patients admitted to the hospital who were asymptomatic, given that many had been counted as Covid admissions.

The CDC needs to shore up its data gathering capacity if we are to be better prepared for the next pandemic.

IN *A TALE OF TWO CITIES*, a book published in 1859 about the French Revolution, Charles Dickens wrote, "It was the best of times, it was the worst of times, it was the age of wisdom, it was the age of foolishness ..." Such was the case with the Covid pandemic.

On the one hand, science saved lives. Eleven months after identifying the virus, the United States had performed two large clinical trials using a novel vaccine strategy, producing vaccines that were remarkably safe and effective. Then it determined how to mass-produce, mass-distribute, and mass-administer them for free, without a preexisting infrastructure for mass-vaccinating adults in place. Covid vaccines were estimated to have saved at least 3.2 million lives. These accomplishments offer hope for how quickly we can respond to the next pandemic.

On the other hand, public health officials had inadvertently leaned into a libertarian left hook. At least 30 states have now passed laws limiting health authorities from imposing protective measures without permission from state legislators. "The courts are leaving us vulnerable," says Wendy Parmet, director of Northwestern University's Center for Health Policy and the Law.

When the next pandemic hits:

• California, Connecticut, Delaware, Florida, Georgia, Louisiana, Montana, New Mexico, New York, North Carolina, North Dakota, Ohio, Oklahoma, South Carolina, and West Virginia will prohibit state governments, schools, and businesses from mandating masks.

- Arizona, Arkansas, Georgia, Florida, Indiana, Montana, New Hampshire, North Dakota, Oklahoma, Tennessee, Texas, and Utah will prohibit state public health agencies from mandating vaccines.

- Health officials in Ohio won't be able to shutter businesses or schools, even if they are the epicenter of an outbreak. Nor will they be able to enforce quarantines, a staple of public health.

- The CDC, handcuffed by a ruling from one judge in Florida, will not be allowed to mandate masks for travel.

- According to a March 2023 ruling by a Texas judge, the president will not be allowed to mandate a vaccine for federal employees.

"One day we're going to have a really bad global crisis and a pandemic far worse than Covid, and we'll look to the government to protect us, but it'll have its hands behind its back and a blindfold on," said Lawrence Gostin, director of Georgetown University's O'Neill Institute for National and Global Health Law. "We'll die with our rights on—we want liberty, but we don't want protection."

ON SUNDAY, DECEMBER 7, 1941, a little before 8:00 a.m., a surprise attack by the Japanese military at Pearl Harbor in Honolulu, Hawaii, killed 2,400 servicemen, ushering in America's involvement in World War II. Americans pulled together, working as one: victory gardens, charity drives, Rosie the Riveter, a large volunteer army. More than 400,000 American soldiers lost their lives to defend this country. We all grieved this shared national tragedy. But we were in it together.

On April 12, 1955, Thomas Francis, standing at the podium in Rackham Hall at the University of Michigan, declared a newly tested polio vaccine to be "safe, potent, and effective." During the 1940s and 1950s, polio was a feared and devastating infection. Americans responded by sending their dimes to the National Foundation for Infantile Paralysis, otherwise known as the March of Dimes. Americans donated millions of dollars to that organization, which led to a vaccine that eventually eliminated polio from most of the world. We made this vaccine. We did this. We saw polio for what it was—another shared national tragedy—and we responded.

On September 11, 2001, two planes hijacked by Islamic jihadists plowed into both towers at the World Trade Center in New York City, killing 2,977 people. Police and firefighters rushed into the collapsing buildings trying to save lives. We all hugged each other and cried, once again united by a shared national tragedy. To further unite us, President George W. Bush made it clear that this event had nothing to do with Muslim Americans. "The face of terror is not the true faith of Islam," he said. "That's not what Islam is all about. Islam is peace. These terrorists don't represent peace." Again, we were all in this together.

On January 20, 2020, the first case of SARS-CoV-2 occurred in the United States. During the next three years, more than a million Americans would lose their lives to this infection. Using a novel technology, we created safe and effective vaccines in record time. Even without proper personal protective equipment, nurses and doctors worked extra hours. It was all hands on deck. People like Ala Stanford, using her own money, tested and vaccinated tens of thousands of residents in an underserved area in North Philadelphia. Again, we responded to a national tragedy. We saw ourselves as part of a whole.

It's in us. We can do this. When we see ourselves as part of something greater, we tap into the better angels of our nature.

In this book, I have told the story of the 2020–23 Covid pandemic. How will we write the story of the next one?

ACKNOWLEDGMENTS

I want to acknowledge the following for their help with this book: Hamid Bassiri, Hilary Black, Brian Fisher, Daniel Griffin, Lori Handy, T. J. Kelleher, Charlotte Moser, Sean O'Connor, Bonnie Offit, Carl Offit, Emily Offit O'Connor, Shannon O'Neill, Dorit Rubinstein Reiss, Gail Ross, and Bambi Short.

SELECTED BIBLIOGRAPHY

INTRODUCTION

Klaassen, F., M. H. Chitwood, T. Cohen et al. "Changes in Population Immunity Against Infection and Severe Disease from SARS-CoV-2 Omicron Variants in the United States Between December 2021 and November 2022." medRxiv (preprint), November 23, 2022. doi.org/10.1101/2022.11.19.22282525.

Little, D., E. Barkley, J. Kibitel et al. "Which Comorbidities Increase the Risk of a Covid-19 Breakthrough Infection." EpicResearch.org, March 31, 2022. epicresearch.org/articles/which-comorbidities-increase-the-risk-of-a-covid-19-breakthrough-infection.

Mandavilli, A. "The CDC Is Not Publishing Large Portions of the Covid Data It Collects." *New York Times*, February 22, 2022.

Stulpin, C. "Universal Masking No Longer Recommended in Health Care Facilities, CDC Says." *Infectious Disease News*, September 30, 2022.

Tin, A. "More Than 9 in 10 Kids Have Survived at Least One Bout with Covid, the CDC Estimates." CBS News, December 15, 2022.

Trinkl, J., K. Bartelt, B. Joyce et al. "Paxlovid Significantly Reduces Covid-19 Hospitalizations and Deaths." EpicResearch.org, September 22, 2022. epicresearch.org/articles/paxlovid-significantly-reduces-covid-19-hospitalizations-and-deaths.

Wen, L. "Public Health Needs a Reset." *Washington Post*, March 7, 2023.

CHAPTER 1:
THE ORIGIN OF A NIGHTMARE

Andersen, K. G., A. Rambaut, W. I. Lipkin et al. "The Proximal Origin of SARS-CoV-2." *Nature Medicine* 26, no. 4 (2020): 450–55.

Cohen, J. "New Clues to Pandemic's Origin Surface, Causing Uproar." *Science* 379, no. 6638 (2023): 1175–76.

Doucleff, M. "What Does the Science Say About the Origin of the SARS-CoV-2 Pandemic." NPR, February 28, 2023.

Dwyer, D. "Watch: Anthony Fauci and Rand Paul Clash Over Wuhan Lab, Origin of Covid-19." Boston.com, May 12, 2021.

Engber, D. "The Lab-Leak Theory Meets Its Perfect Match." *The Atlantic*, November 24, 2021.

Gale, J. "Bats in Laos Caves Harbor Closest Relatives to Covid-19 Virus." Bloomberg, September 18, 2021.

Gordon, M. R., and W. P. Strobel. "Lab Leak Most Likely Origin of Covid-19 Pandemic, Energy Department Now Says." *Wall Street Journal*, February 26, 2023.

Gostin, L. O., and G. K. Gronvall. "The Origins of Covid-19—Why It Matters (and Why It Doesn't)." *New England Journal of Medicine* (2023). doi.org/10.1056/NEJMp2305081.

Graham-Harrison E., T. Phillips, and J. McCurry. "Doctor Who Blew Whistle Over Coronavirus Has Died, Hospital Says." *The Guardian*, February 6, 2020.

Gronvall, G. K. "The Contested Origin of SARS-CoV-2." *Survival* 63, no. 6 (2021): 7–36.

Holmes, E. C., S. A. Goldstein, A. L. Rasmussen et al. "The Origins of SARS-CoV-2: A Critical Review." *Cell* 184, no. 19 (2021): 4848–56.

Honigsbaum, M. "Viral by Alina Chan and Matt Ridley Review—Was Covid-19 Really Made in China?" *The Guardian*, November 15, 2021.

Hu, B., L.-P. Zeng, X.-L. Yang et al. "Discovery of a Rich Gene Pool of Bat SARS-Related Coronaviruses Provides New Insights into the Origin of SARS Coronavirus." *PLOS Pathogenesis* 13, no. 11 (2017). doi.org/10.1371/journal.ppat.1006698.

Kessler, G. "Fact-Checking the Paul-Fauci Flap Over Wuhan Lab Funding." *Washington Post*, May 18, 2021.

Lewis, T. "New Evidence Supports Animal Origin of Covid Virus Through Raccoon Dogs." *Scientific American*, March 17, 2023.

Madhusoodanan, J. "Animal Reservoirs—Where the Next SARS-CoV-2 Variant Could Arise." *Journal of the American Medical Association* 328, no. 8 (2022): 696–98.

Matza, M., and N. Yong. "FBI Chief Christopher Wray Says China Lab Leak Most Likely." BBC.com, March 1, 2023. bbc.com/news/world-us-canada-64806903.

Menachery, V. D., B. L. Yount, Jr., K. Debbink et al. "A SARS-Like Cluster of Circulating Bat Coronaviruses Shows Potential for Human Emergence." *Nature Medicine* 21, no. 12 (2015): 1508–1513.

Mikkelson, D. "AIDS Created by the CIA?" Snopes.com, March 5, 2003 (updated September 22, 2014).

Mueller, B. "New Data Links Pandemic's Origins to Raccoon Dogs at Wuhan Market." *New York Times*, March 16, 2023.

Newey, S. "Chinese Scientists Find 'Suspicious' Feature of Coronavirus in the Wild." *The Telegraph*, May 9, 2023.

"Nobel Peace Laureate Claims HIV Deliberately Created." ABC News, Australia, October 9, 2004. abc.net.au/news/2004-10-09/nobel-peace-laureate-claims-hiv-deliberately/565752.

Pezenik, S., J. Margolin, K. Morris, and T. Moran. "New Report from Senate Republicans Doubles Down on Covid Lab Leak Theory." ABC News, April 18, 2023.

Phillips, A. "'No-Brainer' Covid Was Made in a Lab, Johns Hopkins Doctor Says." *Newsweek*, March 1, 2023.

Quammen, D. *Spillover: Animal Infections and the Next Human Pandemic*, New York: W.W. Norton & Company, 2012.

Rasmussen, A., and M. Worobey. "Covid-19 Almost Certainly Did Not Come from a Lab Leak. Here's How We Know." *Globe and Mail*, July 28, 2022.

Sanders, L., and K. Frankovic. "Two-Thirds of Americans Believe That the Covid-19 Virus Originated from a Lab in China." YouGov America, March 10, 2023.

Worobey, M. "Dissecting the Early Covid-19 Cases in Wuhan." *Science* 374, no. 6572 (2021): 1202–1204.

Worobey, M. "I Called for More Research on the Covid 'Lab Leak Theory.' Here's What I Found." *Los Angeles Times*, March 8, 2023.

Worobey, M., J. I. Levy, L. M. Serrano et al. "The Huanan Seafood Wholesale Market in Wuhan Was the Early Epicenter of the Covid-19 Pandemic." *Science* 377, no. 6609 (2022): 951–59.

Wu, K. "The Strongest Evidence Yet That an Animal Started the Pandemic." *The Atlantic*, March 16, 2023.

Zhu, W., Y. Huang, J. Gong et al. "A Novel Bat Coronavirus with a Polybasic Furin-Like Cleavage Site." *Virologica Sinica* 38, no. 3 (2023): 344–50. doi.org/10.1016/j.virs.2023.04.009.

Zimmer, C. "Newly Discovered Bat Viruses Give Hints to Covid's Origins." *New York Times*, October 14, 2021.

CHAPTER 2: THE LURE OF CONSPIRACY

Andrews, T. "Facebook and Other Companies Are Removing Viral 'Plandemic' Conspiracy Video." *Washington Post*, May 7, 2020.

Cook, J., S. van der Linden, S. Lewandowsky, and U. Ecker. "Coronavirus, 'Plandemic' and the Seven Traits of Conspiratorial Thinking." *The Conversation*, May 15, 2020.

Darby, L. "What Is 'Plandemic,' the Latest Anti-Vaxxer Conspiracy Theory?" *GQ*, May 11, 2020.

Enserink, M., and J. Cohen. "Fact-Checking Judy Mikovits, the Controversial Virologist Attacking Anthony Fauci in a Viral Conspiracy Video." *Science*, May 8, 2020.

Fichera, A., S. H. Spencer, D. Gore, L. Robertson, and E. Kiely. "The Falsehoods of the 'Plandemic' Video." FactCheck.org, May 8, 2020 (updated June 29, 2021).

Frenkel, S., B. Decker, and D. Alba. "How the 'Plandemic' Movie and Its Falsehoods Spread Widely Online." *New York Times*, May 20, 2020.

Funke, D. "Fact-Checking 'Plandemic': A Documentary Full of False Conspiracy Theories About the Coronavirus." *Politifact*, May 7, 2020.

Haelle, T. "Why It's Important to Push Back on 'Plandemic'—And How to Do It." *Forbes*, May 8, 2020.

"The Infodemic: *Plandemic 2* Is Another Covid-19 Conspiracy Theory Video." Voice of America, August 19, 2020.

Kearney, M. D., S. C. Chiang, and P. M. Massey. "The Twitter Origins and Evolution of the Covid-19 'Plandemic' Conspiracy Theory." *Misinformation Review*, Harvard Kennedy School, October 9, 2020.

Landsverk, G., and A. Woodward. "A Point-By-Point Debunk of the 'Plandemic' Movie, Which Was Shared Widely Before YouTube and Facebook Took It Down." *Business Insider*, May 22, 2020.

"Millions View Viral Plandemic Video Featuring Discredited Medical Researcher Judy Mikovits." ABC/Reuters, May 13, 2020.

Naughton, J. "How the 'Plandemic' Conspiracy Theory Took Hold." *The Guardian,* May 23, 2020.

Nazar, S., and T. Pieters. "Plandemic Revisited: A Product of Planned Disinformation Amplifying the Covid-19 'Infodemic.'" *Frontiers in Public Health* 9 (July 14, 2021). doi.org/10.3389/fpubh.2021.649930.

Neuman, S. "Seen 'Plandemic'? We Take a Close Look at the Viral Conspiracy Video's Claims." NPR, May 8, 2020.

Sommer, W. "Discredited Doctor and Sham 'Science' Are the Stars of Viral Coronavirus Documentary 'Plandemic.'" *Daily Beast,* May 8, 2020.

Spencer, S. H., J. McDonald, and A. Fichera. "New 'Plandemic' Video Peddles Misinformation, Conspiracies." FactCheck.org, August 21, 2020 (updated June 29, 2021).

Spring, M. "Coronavirus: 'Plandemic' Virus Conspiracy Video Spreads Across Social Media." BBC News, May 8, 2020.

Trang, B. "Covid Vaccines Averted 3 Million Deaths in U.S., According to New Study." *STAT,* December 13, 2022.

Zadrozny, B., and B. Collins. "As '#Plandemic' Goes Viral, Those Targeted by Discredited Scientist's Crusade Warn of 'Dangerous' Claims." NBC News, May 7, 2020.

CHAPTER 3: THE FDA STUMBLES

HYDROXYCHLOROQUINE

Aljadeed, R. "The Rise and Fall of Hydroxychloroquine and Chloroquine in Covid-19." *Journal of Pharmacy Practice* 35, no. 6 (2021): 971–78.

Axfors, C., A. M. Schmitt, P. Janiaud et al. "Mortality Outcomes with Hydroxychloroquine and Chloroquine in Covid-19 from an International Collaborative Meta-Analysis of Randomized Trials." *Nature Communications* 12, no. 2349 (2021). doi.org/10.1038/s41467-021-22446-z.

Bansal, P., A. Goyal, A. Cusick IV et al. "Hydroxychloroquine: A Comprehensive Review and Its Controversial Role in Coronavirus Disease 2019." *Annals of Medicine* 53, no. 1 (2020): 117–34.

Barratt-Due, A., I. C. Olsen, K. Nezvalova-Henriksen et al. "Evaluation of the Effects of Remdesivir and Hydroxychloroquine on Viral Clearance in Covid-19." *Annals of Internal Medicine* 174, no. 9 (2021): 1261–69.

Benen, S. "Trump Thinks He May Have 'A Natural Ability' to Address Viral Outbreaks." MSNBC, March 9, 2020.

Cavalcanti, A. B., R. G. Zampieri, R. G. Rosa et al. "Hydroxychloroquine With or Without Azithromycin in Mild-to-Moderate Covid-19." *New England Journal of Medicine* 383 (2020): 2041–52.

Ferner, R. E., and J. K. Aronson. "Chloroquine and Hydroxychloroquine in Covid-19." *British Medical Journal* 369 (2020). doi.org/10.1136/bmj .m1432.

Fiolet, T., A. Guihur, M. E. Rebeaud et al. "Effect of Hydroxychloroquine With or Without Azithromycin on the Mortality of Coronavirus Disease 2019 (Covid-19) Patients: A Systematic Review and Meta-Analysis." *Clinical Microbiology and Infection* 27, no. 1 (2021): 19–27.

Gautret, P., J.-C. Lagier, P. Parola et al. "Hydroxychloroquine and Azithromycin as a Treatment of Covid-19: Results of an Open-Label Non-Randomized Clinical Trial." *International Journal of Antimicrobial Agents* 56, no. 1 (2020). doi.org/10.1016 /j.ijantimicag.2020.105949.

Ghazy, R. M., A. Almaghraby, R. Shaaban et al. "A Systematic Review and Meta-Analysis on Chloroquine and Hydroxychloroquine as Monotherapy or Combined with Azithromycin in Covid-19 Treatment." *Scientific Reports* 10, no. 22139 (2020). doi.org/10.1038/s41598-020-77748-x.

Hoffman, M., K. Mösbauer, H. Hofmann-Winkler et al. "Chloroquine Does Not Inhibit Infection of Human Lung Cells with SARS-CoV-2." *Nature* 585, no. 7826 (2020): 588–90.

Hussain, N., E. Chung, J. J. Heyl et al. "A Meta-Analysis on the Effects of Hydroxychloroquine on Covid-19." *Cureus* 12, no. 8 (2020). doi.org/10.7759/ cureus.10005.

Ip, A., J. Ahn, Y. Zhou et al. "Hydroxychloroquine in the Treatment of Outpatients with Mildly Symptomatic Covid-19: A Multi-Center Observational Study." *BMC Infectious Diseases* 21, no. 1 (2021): 72. doi.org/10.1186/s12879-021-05773-w.

Lewis, K., D. Chaudhuri, F. Alshamsi et al. "The Efficacy and Safety of Hydroxychloroquine for Covid-19 Prophylaxis: A Systematic Review and Meta-Analysis of Randomized Trials." *PLOS ONE* 16, no. 1 (2021): e0244778. doi.org/10.1371/journal .pone.0244778.

Liu, J., R. Cao, M. Xu et al. "Hydroxychloroquine, a Less Toxic Derivative of Chloroquine, Is Effective in Inhibiting SARS-CoV-2 Infection In Vitro." *Cell Discovery* 6, no. 16 (2020). doi.org/10.1038/ s41421-020-0156-0.

Mahase, E. "Hydroxychloroquine for Covid-19: The End of the Line?" *British Medical Journal* 369 (2020): m2378. doi.org/10.1136/bmj.m2378.

Maisonnasse, P., J. Guedj, V. Contreras et al. "Hydroxychloroquine Use Against SARS-CoV-2 Infection in Non-Human Primates." *Nature* 585, no. 7826 (2020): 584–87.

Manivannan, E., C. Karthikeyan, N. S. Hari Narayana Moorthy et al. "The Rise and Fall of Chloroquine/Hydroxychloroquine as Compassionate Therapy of Covid-19." *Frontiers in Pharmacology* 12 (2021): 584940. doi.org/10.3389/fphar.2021.584940.

Martins-Filho, R. R., L. C. Ferreira, L. Heimfarth et al. "Efficacy and Safety of Hydroxychloroquine as Pre- and Post-Exposure Prophylaxis and Treatment of Covid-19: A Systematic Review and Meta-Analysis of Blinded, Placebo-Controlled, Randomized Clinical Trails." *Lancet Regional Health—Americas* 2, no. 100062 (2021). doi.org/10.1016/j.lana.2021.100062.

RECOVERY Collaborative Group. "Effect of Hydroxychloroquine in Hospitalized Patients with Covid-19." *New England Journal of Medicine* 383, no. 21 (2020): 2030–40.

Saag, M. S. "Misguided Use of Hydroxychloroquine for Covid-19." *Journal of the American Medical Association* 324, no. 21 (2020): 2161–62.

Sayare, S. "He Was a Science Star. Then He Promoted a Questionable Cure for Covid-19." *New York Times*, May 12, 2020 (updated May 21, 2020).

Self, W. H., M. W. Semler, L. M. Leither et al. "Effect of Hydroxychloroquine on Clinical Status at 14 Days in Hospitalized Patients with Covid-19: A Randomized Clinical Trial." *Journal of the American Medical Association* 324, no. 21 (2020): 2165–76.

Sivapalan, P., C. S. Ulrik, T. S. Lapperre et al. "Azithromycin and Hydroxychloroquine in Hospitalised Patients with Confirmed Covid-19: A Randomised Double-Blinded Placebo-Controlled Trial." *European Respiratory Journal* (2022). doi.org/10.1183/13993003.00752-2021.

Takla, M., and K. Jeevaratnam. "Chloroquine, Hydroxychloroquine, and Covid-19: Systematic Review and Narrative Synthesis of Efficacy and Safety." *Saudi Pharmaceutical Journal* 28, no. 12 (2020): 1760–76.

WHO Solidarity Trial Consortium et al. "Repurposed Antiviral Drugs for Covid-19—Interim WHO Solidarity Trial Results." *New England Journal of Medicine* 384 (2021): 497–511.

Xu, J., and B. Cao. "Lessons Learnt from Hydroxychloroquine/Azithromycin in Treatment of Covid-19." *European Respiratory Journal* 59 (2021): 2102002. doi.org/10.1183/13993003.02002-2021.

CONVALESCENT PLASMA

Agarwal, A., A. Mukherjee, G. Kumar et al. "Convalescent Plasma in the Management of Moderate Covid-19 in Adults in India: Open Label Phase II Multicentre Randomised Controlled Trial (PLACID Trial)." *British Medical Journal* 371 (2020): m3939.

Agarwal, N., S. Mishra, and A. Ayub. "Convalescent Plasma Therapy in Covid-19 and Discharge Status: A Systematic Review." *Journal of Family Medicine and Primary Care* 10, no. 10 (2021): 3876–81.

Alsharidah, S., M. Ayed, R. M. Ameen et al. "Covid-19 Convalescent Plasma Treatment of Moderate and Severe Cases of SARS-CoV-2 Infection: A Multicenter Interventional Study." *International Journal of Infectious Diseases* 103 (2021): 439–46.

Axfors, C. P. Janiaud, A. M. Schmitt et al. "Association Between Convalescent Plasma Treatment and Mortality in Covid-19: A Collaborative Systematic Review and Meta-Analysis of Randomized Clinical Trials." *BMC Infectious Diseases* 21, no. 1170 (2021). doi.org/10.1186/s12879-021-06829-7.

Bégin, P., J. Callum, E. Jamula et al. "Convalescent Plasma for Hospitalized Patients with Covid-19: An Open-Label, Randomized Controlled Trial." *Nature Medicine* 27, no. 11 (2021): 2012–24.

Casadevall, A., Q. Dragotakes, P. W. Johnson et al. "Convalescent Plasma Use in the USA Was Inversely Correlated with Covid-19 Mortality." *eLife* 10, no. e69866 (2021). doi.org/10.7554/eLife.69866.

Cho, K., S. C. Keithly, K. E. Kurgansky et al. "Early Convalescent Plasma Therapy and Mortality Among US Veterans Hospitalized with Nonsevere Covid-19: An Observational Analysis Emulating a Target Trial." *Journal of Infectious Diseases* 224, no. 6 (2021): 967–75.

Duan, K., B. Liu, C. Li et al. "Effectiveness of Convalescent Plasma Therapy in Severe Covid-19 Patients." *Proceedings of the National Academy of Sciences* 117, no. 17 (2020): 9490–96.

Elbadawi, A., M. Shnoda, M. Laguio-Vila et al. "Convalescent Plasma in the Management of Covid-19 Pneumonia." *European Journal of Internal Medicine* 89 (2021): 121–23.

Hatzl, S., F. Posch, N. Sareban et al. "Convalescent Plasma Therapy and Mortality in Covid-19 Patients Admitted to the ICU: A Prospective Observational Study." *Annals of Intensive Care* 11, no. 1 (2021): 73. doi.org/10.1186/s13613-021-00867-9.

Joyner, M. J., J. W. Senefeld, S. A. Klassen et al. "Effect

Selected Bibliography

of Convalescent Plasma on Mortality Among Hospitalized Patients with Covid-19: Initial Three-Month Experience." medRxiv (2020). doi.org/10.1101/2020.08.12.20169359.

Klassen, S. A., J. W. Senefeld, P. W. Johnson et al. "The Effect of Convalescent Plasma Therapy on Mortality Among Patients with Covid-19: Systematic Review and Meta-Analysis." *Mayo Clinic Proceedings* 96, no. 5 (2021): 1262–75.

Klassen, S. A., J. W. Senefeld, K. A. Senese et al. "Convalescent Plasma Therapy for Covid-19: A Graphical Mosaic of the Worldwide Evidence." *Frontiers in Medicine* 8 (2021). doi.org/10.3389/fmed.2021.684151.

Kloypan, C., M. Saesong, J. Sangsuemoon et al. "Convalescent Plasma for Covid-19: A Meta-Analysis of Clinical Trials and Real-World Evidence." *European Journal of Clinical Investigation* 51, no. 11 (2021): e13663. doi.org/10.1111/eci.13663.

Korley, F. K., V. Durkalski-Mauldin, S. D. Yeatts et al. "Early Convalescent Plasma for High-Risk Outpatients with Covid-19." *New England Journal of Medicine* 385, no. 21 (2021): 1951–60.

Lattanzio, N., C. Acosta-Diaz, R. J. Villasmil et al. "Effectiveness of Covid-19 Convalescent Plasma Infusion Within 48 Hours of Hospitalization with SARS-CoV-2 Infection." *Cureus* 13, no. 7 (2021): e16746. doi.org/10.7759/cureus.16746.

Mucha, S. R., and N. Quraishy. "Convalescent Plasma for Covid-19: Promising, Not Proven." *Cleveland Clinic Journal of Medicine* 87, no. 11 (2020): 664–70.

Peng, H. T., S. G. Rhind, and A. Beckett. "Convalescent Plasma for the Prevention and Treatment of Covid-19: A Systematic Review and Quantitative Analysis." *JMIR Public Health and Surveillance* 7, no. 6 (2021): e31554. doi.org/10.2196/25500.

Piscoya, A., L. F. Ng-Sueng, A. P. del Riego et al. "Efficacy and Harms of Convalescent Plasma for Treatment of Hospitalized Covid-19 Patients: A Systematic Review and Meta-Analysis." *Archives of Medical Science* 17, no. 5 (2021): 1251–61.

Salazar, E., K. K. Perez, M. Ashraf et al. "Treatment of Coronavirus Disease 2019 (Covid-19) Patients with Convalescent Plasma." *American Journal of Pathology* 190, no. 8 (2020): 1680–90.

Salman, O. H., and H. S. A. Mohamed. "Efficacy and Safety of Transfusing Plasma from Covid-19 Survivors to Covid-19 Victims with Severe Illness: A Double-Blinded Controlled Preliminary Study." *Egyptian Journal of Anaesthesia* 36, no. 1 (2020): 264–72.

Sekine, L., B. Arns, B. R. Fabro et al. "Convalescent Plasma for Covid-19 in Hospitalised Patients: An Open-Label, Randomised Clinical Trial." *European Respiratory Journal* 59, no. 2 (2021): 2101471. doi.org/10.1183/13993003.01471-2021.

Simonovich, V. A., L. D. Pratx, P. Scibona et al. "A Randomized Trial of Convalescent Plasma in Covid-19 Severe Pneumonia." *New England Journal of Medicine* 384, no. 7 (2021): 619–29.

Sullivan, D. J., K. A. Gebo, S. Shoham et al. "Early Outpatient Treatment for Covid-19 with Convalescent Plasma." *New England Journal of Medicine* 386, no. 18 (2022): 1700-1711.

Tortosa, F., G. Carrasco, M. Ragusa et al. "Use of Convalescent Plasma in Patients with Coronavirus Disease (Covid-19): Systematic Review and Meta-Analysis." medRxiv (preprint). doi.org/10.1101/2021.02.14.20246454.

Wooding, D. J., and H. Bach. "Treatment of Covid-19 with Convalescent Plasma: Lessons from Past Coronavirus Outbreaks." *Clinical Microbiology and Infection* 26, no. 10 (2020): 1436–46.

Writing Committee for the REMAP-CAP Investigators. "Effect of Convalescent Plasma on Organ Support-Free Days in Critically Ill Patients with Covid-19: A Randomized Clinical Trial." *Journal of the American Medical Association* 326, no. 17 (2021): 1690–1702.

STEPHEN HAHN

Baumann, J. "Botched Covid Plasma Announcement Clouds FDA's Vaccine Process." *Bloomberg Law*, August 25, 2020.

Blake, A. "The FDA Offers a Big Correction After Helping Hype Trump's Coronavirus Announcement." *Washington Post*, August 24, 2020.

Carr, T. "Is the Trump Administration Eroding Trust in the FDA?" *Undark*, October 14, 2020.

"Coronavirus (Covid-19) Update: FDA Encourages Recovered Patients to Donate Plasma for Development of Blood-Related Therapies." U.S. Food and Drug Administration, April 16, 2020.

Edwards, E. "Why Did the FDA Authorize Convalescent Plasma, a Potential Treatment for Covid-19?" NBC News, August 24, 2020.

"FDA Chief Apologizes for Overstating Plasma Effect on Virus." Associated Press, August 25, 2020.

"FDA Issues Emergency Use Authorization for Convalescent Plasma as Potential Promising Covid-19 Treatment, Another Achievement in Administration's Fight Against Pandemic." U.S. Food and Drug Administration, August 23, 2020.

Florka, N. "FDA, Under Pressure from Trump, Authorizes Blood Plasma as Covid-19 Treatment." *STAT,* August 23, 2020.

Hiltzik, M. "Column: FDA Boss Hahn Admits Error on Plasma, But Fails to Recover His Credibility." *Los Angeles Times,* August 25, 2020.

Kinch, M. S., and J. P. Henderson. "How Politics Muddied the Waters on a Promising Covid-19 Treatment." *Scientific American,* August 25, 2020.

Kupferschmidt, K., and J. Cohen. "In FDA's Green Light for Treating Covid-19 with Plasma, Critics See Thin Evidence—and Politics." *Science,* August 24, 2020.

Oprysko, C. "FDA Chief Issues Mea Culpa for His Plasma Treatment Claims." *Politico,* August 25, 2020.

"President Trump News Conference." C-SPAN, August 23, 2020.

Rutschman, A. S., L. Vertinsky, and Y. Heled. "Opinion: We Worry the FDA Is Under Extreme Pressure to Rush Approvals for Covid-19 Treatments." *Market Watch,* August 27, 2020.

Rutschman, A., L. Vertinsky, and Y. Heled. "FDA Is Departing from Long-Standing Procedures to Deal with Public Health Crises, and This May Foreshadow Problems for Covid-19 Vaccines." *The Conversation,* August 27, 2020.

Sachs, R. "Understanding the FDA's Controversial Convalescent Plasma Authorization." *Health Affairs,* August 27, 2020.

Sharfstein, J. "How the FDA Should Protect Its Integrity from Politics." *Nature,* September 9, 2020.

Thomas, K., and S. Fink. "F.D.A. 'Grossly Misrepresented' Blood Plasma Data, Scientists Say." *New York Times,* August 24, 2020.

CHAPTER 4: A TICKET OUT

Gargano, J. W., M. Wallace, S. C. Hadler et al. "Use of mRNA Covid-19 Vaccine After Reports of Myocarditis Among Vaccine Recipients: Update from the Advisory Committee on Immunization Practices—United States, June 2021." *Morbidity and Mortality Weekly Report* 70, no. 27 (July 9, 2021).

Hahn, S. M. "Opinion: FDA Commissioner: No Matter What, Only a Safe, Effective Vaccine Will Get Our Approval." *Washington Post,* August 5, 2020.

Islam, A., M. S. Bashir, K. Joyce et al. "An Update on Covid-19 Vaccine Induced Thrombotic Thrombocytopenia Syndrome and Some Management Recommendations." *Molecule* 26, no. 16 (August 18, 2021).

Knight, R., V. Walker, S. Ip et al. "Association of Covid-19 with Major Arterial and Venous Thrombotic Diseases: A Population-Wide Cohort Study of 48 Million Adults in England and Wales." *Circulation* 146, no. 12 (2022): 892–906.

Mostafavi, A., S. A. H. Tabatabaei, S. Z. Fard et al. "The Incidence of Myopericarditis in Patients with Covid-19." *Journal of Cardiovascular Thoracic Research* 13, no. 3 (2021): 203–207.

Offit, P. A. *Vaccinated: One Man's Quest to Defeat the World's Deadliest Diseases.* New York: HarperCollins, 2007.

"Operation Warp Speed: Accelerated Covid-19 Vaccine Development Status and Efforts to Address Manufacturing Challenges." Government Accounting Office, February 2021.

Watanabe, A., R. Kani, M. Iwagami et al. "Assessment of Efficacy and Safety of mRNA Covid-19 Vaccines in Children Aged 5 to 11 Years: A Systematic Review and Meta-Analysis." *Journal of the American Medicine Association Pediatrics* 177, no. 4 (2023). doi.org/10.1001/jamapediatrics.2022.6243.

Yasuhara, J., K. Masuda, T. Aikawa et al. "Myopericarditis After Covid-19 mRNA Vaccination Among Adolescents and Young Adults: A Systematic Review and Meta-Analysis." *Journal of the American Medicine Association Pediatrics* 177, no. 1 (2022). doi.org/10.1001/jamapediatrics.2022.4768.

CHAPTER 5:
THE MISINFORMATION BUSINESS

Alba, D. "YouTube Bans All Anti-Vaccine Misinformation." *New York Times,* September 29, 2021.

Basen, R. "Doc Fired After Standing Up to Private Equity: RFK Jr.'s Anti-Vax Machine." *MedPage Today,* December 21, 2021.

Bradner, E., and K. Maher. "DeSantis Targets Covid Vaccine Manufacturers and CDC in Latest Anti-Vaccine Moves." CNN, December 13, 2022.

Brashier, N., G. Pennycook, A. J. Berinsky et al. "Timing Matters When Correcting Fake News." *Proceedings of the National Academy of Sciences* 118, no. 5 (2021). doi.org/10.1073/pnas.2020043118.

Bredderman, W. "How a Clinton Associate Bankrolled the Anti-Vax Underground." *Daily Beast,* October 29, 2021.

Brumfiel, G. "For Some Anti-Vaccine Advocates, Misinformation Is Part of a Business." NPR, May 12, 2021.

Brumfiel, G. "Anti-Vaccine Activists Use a Federal Database to Spread Fear About Covid Vaccines." NPR, June 14, 2021.

Selected Bibliography

Center for Countering Digital Hate. *The Disinformation Dozen: Why Platforms Must Act on Twelve Leading Online Anti-Vaxxers*, March 24, 2021. counterhate.com/disinformationdozen.

Dean, J., and G. Duff. "Joe Mercola: An Antivaccine Quack Tycoon Pivots Effortlessly to Profit from Spreading Covid-19 Misinformation." *Veterans Today*, August 6, 2021.

Devine, C., and D. Griffin. "Leaders of the Anti-Vaccine Movement Used 'Stop the Steal' Crusade to Advance Their Own Conspiracy Theories." CNN, February 5, 2021.

Dvorak, P. "The Anti-Vaxxers Are Coming to D.C., and Their Leader Is a Kennedy." *Washington Post*, January 20, 2022.

Frenkel, S. "The Most Influential Spreader of Coronavirus Misinformation Online." *New York Times*, July 24, 2021.

Gorski, D. "Joe Mercola: Quackery Pays." *Science-Based Medicine*, February 6, 2012.

Haelle, T. "This Is the Moment the Anti-Vaccine Movement Has Been Waiting For." *New York Times*, August 31, 2021.

Hiltzik, M. "Column: Following FDA Approval of Pfizer's Shot, the Anti-Vaccine Movement Cooks Up New Conspiracy Theory." *Los Angeles Times*, September 1, 2021.

Jamison, P., and E. Silverman. "Anti-Vaccine Activists See D.C. Rally as a Marker of Recent Gains." *Washington Post*, January 22, 2022.

Kakkar, H., and A. Lawson. "We Found the One Group of Americans Who Are Most Likely to Spread Fake News." *Politico*, January 14, 2022.

Kolata, G. "Tucker Carlson Has a Cure for Declining Virility." *New York Times*, April 22, 2022.

Krugman, P. "The Snake Oil Theory of the Modern Right." *New York Times*, August 30, 2021.

Kunzelman, M. "Anti-Vaccine Doctor Sentenced to Prison for Capitol Riot." Associated Press, June 16, 2022.

Lawson, M. A., and H. Kakkar. "Of Pandemics, Politics, and Personality: The Role of Conscientiousness and Political Ideology in the Sharing of Fake News." *Journal of Experimental Psychology, General* 151, no. 5 (2022): 1154–77.

Levitz, E. "Levitz: 'Fox News Is Literally Killing Its Viewers' with Covid Lies." MSNBC, January 26, 2022.

McIntosh, A. M., J. McMahon, L. M. Dibbons et al. "Effects of Vaccination on Onset and Outcome of

Dravet Syndrome: A Retrospective Study." *Lancet Neurology* 9, no. 6 (2010): 593–98.

Nagourney, A. "A Kennedy's Crusade Against Covid Vaccines Anguishes Family and Friends." *New York Times*, February 26, 2022.

Peiser, J. "Miami School Says Vaccinated Students Must Stay Home for 30 Days to Protect Others, Citing Discredited Info." *Washington Post*, October 18, 2021.

Pengelly, M. "Guests Urged to Be Vaccinated at Anti-Vaxxer Robert F Kennedy Jr's Party." *The Guardian*, December 18, 2021.

Rawat, D., A. Roy, S. Maitra et al. "Vitamin C and Covid-19 Treatment: A Systematic Review and Meta-Analysis of Randomized Controlled Trials." *Diabetes & Metabolic Syndrome: Clinical Research & Reviews* 15, no. 6 (2021): 102324.

Reilly, P. "RFK Jr. Says Wife Cheryl Hines, Not Him, Urged Party Guests to Be Vaxxed for Covid." *New York Post*, December 18, 2021.

Reiss, J., and M. R. Smith. "Inside One Network Cashing in on Vaccine Disinformation." AP News, May 13, 2021.

"RFK Jr.'s Anti-Vaccine Group Kicked Off Instagram and Facebook." Associated Press, August 18, 2022.

Riess, R., and G. Lemos. "Miami Private School Makes Bogus Claims About Vaccines While Ordering Pupils Who Get a Shot to Stay Home for 30 Days." CNN, October 19, 2021.

Ross, J. "Anti-Vaxxer Robert F. Kennedy Jr.'s House Party Guests Told to Get Vaccinated Before Coming." *Daily Beast*, December 17, 2021.

Salam, E. "Majority of Covid Misinformation Came From 12 People, Report Finds." *The Guardian*, July 17, 2021.

Shanahan, M., and H. Krueger. "RFK Jr.'s Anti-Vaccine Crusade Deepens Rift with Family and Friends." *Boston Globe*, January 29, 2022.

Smith, M. R. "How a Kennedy Built an Anti-Vaccine Juggernaut Amid Covid-19." AP News, December 15, 2021.

Wadhwani, A. "Former Tennessee Vaccine Chief Fiscus Seeks to Have Name Cleared in Court." *Tennessee Lookout*, December 5, 2022.

Weir, K. "How Robert F. Kennedy Jr. Became the Anti-Vaxxer Icon of America's Nightmares." *Vanity Fair*, May 13, 2021.

Whitehurst, L., A. D. Richer, and M. Kunzelman. "Oath Keepers Founder Stewart Rhodes Convicted of

Seditious Conspiracy in Jan. 6 Case." *Los Angeles Times,* November 29, 2022.

Zadrozny, B. "Once Struggling, Anti-Vaccination Groups Have Enjoyed a Pandemic Windfall." NBC News, February 3, 2022.

CHAPTER 6: ROGUE SCIENTIST: THE REMARKABLE STORY OF ROBERT MALONE

Alba, D. "The Latest Covid Misinformation Star Says He Invented the Vaccines." *New York Times,* April 3, 2022.

Alexander, H. "The Truth About Joe Rogan's Controversial Guests." *Daily Mail,* February 2, 2022.

Bartlett, T. "The Vaccine Scientist Spreading Vaccine Misinformation." *The Atlantic,* August 12, 2021.

Bella, T. "A Vaccine Scientist's Discredited Claims Have Bolstered a Movement of Misinformation." *Washington Post,* January 24, 2022.

Brueck, H. "The Rise of Robert Malone, the mRNA Scientist Turned Vaccine Skeptic Who Shot to Fame on Joe Rogan's Podcast." *Insider,* February 27, 2022.

Daniels, C. J., S. Rajpal, J. T. Greenshields et al. "Prevalence of Clinical and Subclinical Myocarditis in Competitive Athletes with Recent SARS-CoV-2 Infection: Results from the Big Ten Covid-19 Cardiac Registry." *Journal of the American Medical Association Cardiology* 6, no. 9 (2021): 1078–87.

Dolgin, E. "The Tangled History of mRNA Vaccines." *Nature* 597, no. 7876 (2021): 318–24.

"Fact Check: CDC Did Not 'Admit' Covid-19 Can Only Be Caught Once." Reuters Fact Check, Reuters, December 27, 2021.

Hernandez, J. "Spotify Will Add a Covid Advisory to Podcasts After the Joe Rogan Controversy." NPR, January 30, 2022.

Kolata, G., and B. Mueller. "Halting Progress and Happy Accidents: How mRNA Vaccines Were Made." *New York Times,* January 15, 2022.

Kwan, M. Y. W., G. T. Chua, C. B. Chow et al. "mRNA Covid Vaccine and Myocarditis in Adolescents." *Hong Kong Medical Journal* 27, no. 5 (2021): 326–27.

Malone, R. W., P. L. Felgner, and I. M. Verma. "Cationic Liposome-Mediated RNA Transfection." *Proceedings of the National Academy of Science, USA* 86, no. 16 (1989): 6077–81.

Milbank, D. "Opinion: Pro-Lifers, RIP. The Pro-Death Movement Is Born." *Washington Post,* January 24, 2022.

Qui, L. "Fact-Checking Joe Rogan's Interview with Robert Malone that Caused an Uproar." *New York Times,* February 8, 2022.

Warmflash, D. "The (Sort of, Partial) Father of mRNA Vaccines Who Now Spreads Vaccine Misinformation (Parts 1 and 2)." *Health Care Blog,* May 17 and 18, 2022.

Wolff, J. A., R. W. Malone, P. Williams et al. "Direct Gene Transfer into Mouse Muscle in Vivo." *Science* (1990) 247, no. 4949: 1465–68.

CHAPTER 7: A PANDEMIC OF THE UNVACCINATED

Blake, A. "The Most-Vaccinated Big Counties in America Are Beating the Worst of the Coronavirus." *Washington Post,* December 4, 2021.

Block, G. "Popular Journalist and Staunch Anti-Vaxxer Dies of Covid-19." *Stuff,* November 29, 2021.

Brumfiel, G. "Inside the Growing Alliance Between Anti-Vaccine Activists and Pro-Trump Republicans." NPR, December 6, 2021.

Cobia, B. "Dr. Brytney Cobia Talks Her Viral 'I'm Sorry, But It's Too Late' Social Media Post." AL.com, December 24, 2021.

Dawson, B. "Anti-Vaxxer Podcaster Dies from Covid-19 After Contracting Virus at Far-Right ReAwaken America Conference." *Business Insider,* January 8, 2022.

Enten, H. "Flu Shots Uptake Is Now Partisan. It Didn't Use to Be." CNN, November 14, 2021.

Fitzsimons, T. "Anti-Vaccine Christian Broadcaster Marcus Lamb Dies at 64 After Contracting Covid." NBC News, November 30, 2021.

Georgiou, A. "Economist Robin Fransman, a Prominent Coronavirus Vaccine Skeptic, Has Died From Covid." *Newsweek,* December 29, 2021.

Gettys, T. "Anti-Vaxx Nurse Dies from Covid-19 in Louisiana." *Raw Story,* July 12, 2021.

Jena, A. B., and C. M. Worsham. "Facts Alone Aren't Going to Win Over the Unvaccinated. This Might." *New York Times,* December 21, 2021.

Mark, J. "He's Declining a Coronavirus Vaccine at the Expense of a Lifesaving Transplant: 'I Was Born Free, I'll Die Free.'" *Washington Post,* January 31, 2022.

McDuffie, W. "Boston Hospital Denies Heart Transplant to Man Who Hasn't Gotten Covid-19 Vaccine." ABC News, January 26, 2022.

Montgomery, D. "How to Sell the Coronavirus Vaccines to a Divided, Uneasy America." *Washington Post Magazine,* April 26, 2021.

"Naturopath Who Sold Fake Vaccine Cards Gets Nearly 3 Years." Associated Press, November 29, 2022.

"Nearly Half of Nursing Home Workers in Pennsylvania Have Declined Covid-19 Vaccine, State Data Shows." CBS News, 3 Philly, April 19, 2021.

Pillion, D. "'I'm Sorry, But It's Too Late': Alabama Doctor on Treating Unvaccinated, Dying Covid Patients." AL.com, July 21, 2021.

Quinn, A. "Anti-Vax Priest Who Claimed Vaccines Contain 'Aborted Embryos' Dies of Covid." Daily Beast, February 3, 2022.

Smith, A. "A Trio of Conservative Radio Hosts Died of Covid. Will Their Deaths Change Vaccine Resistance?" NBC News, September 3, 2021.

Sommer, W. "QAnon Star Who Said Only 'Idiots' Get Vax Dies of Covid." Daily Beast, January 7, 2022.

Tufekci, Z. "The Unvaccinated May Not Be Who You Think." New York Times, October 15, 2021.

U.S. Attorney's Office, District of South Carolina. "Nursing Director Pleads Guilty to Lying to Federal Agents Regarding Production of Fraudulent Covid-19 Vaccine Cards." June 23, 2022.

"Why Millennials and Gen Z Aren't Getting Vaccinated—And What to Do About It." Advisory Board, April 26, 2021 (updated on May 7, 2021 and March 20, 2023).

ALA STANFORD

McGrath, M. "Dr. Ala Stanford and the Women Who, Ages 50 and Over, Are Leading the Fight Against Covid." Forbes, February 26, 2021.

Muse, Q. "How Ala Stanford Became a Champion for the Health of Black Philadelphians Amid Covid." Philadelphia Magazine, August 8, 2020.

Palmer, S. "Family, Community, and Social Justice Converge in this Eberly Alumna's Medical Practice." Penn State Alumni Magazine, March 9, 2021.

Toner, K. "This CNN Hero Is Fighting to Save Lives in Philadelphia's Communities of Color Through Covid-19 Vaccination and Testing." CNN, June 24, 2021.

Vitarelli, A. "Dr. Ala Stanford Honored with Philadelphia Magazine's 2021 Trailblazer Award." WPVI, July 15, 2021.

CHAPTER 8: BOOSTER CONFUSION: WHO IS PROTECTED?

Agrawal, U., S. Bedston, C. McCowan, et al. "Severe Covid-19 Outcomes After Full Vaccination of Primary Schedule and Initial Boosters: Pooled Analysis of National Prospective Cohort Studies of 30 Million Individuals in England, Northern Ireland, Scotland, and Wales." Lancet 400, no. 10360 (2022): 1305–20.

Auvigne, V., C. Tamandjou, J. Schaeffer et al. "Protection Against Symptomatic SARS-CoV-2 BA.5 Infection Conferred by the Pfizer-BioNTech Original/BA.4-5 Bivalent Vaccine Compared to the mRNA Original (Ancestral) Monovalent Vaccines—A Matched Cohort Study in France." medRxiv (preprints), March 28, 2023. doi.org/10.1101/2023.03.17.23287411.

Bar-On, Y. M., Y. Goldberg, M. Mandel et al. "Protection of BNT162b2 Vaccine Booster Against Covid-19 in Israel." New England Journal of Medicine 385 (2021): 1393–1400.

Bowen, J. E., A. Addetia, H. V. Dang et al. "Omicron Spike Function and Neutralizing Activity Elicited by a Comprehensive Panel of Vaccines." Science 377, no. 6608 (2022): 890–94.

Brown, C. M., J. Vostok, H. Johnson et al. "Outbreak of SARS-CoV-2 Infections, Including Covid-19 Vaccine Breakthrough Infections, Associated with Large Public Gatherings—Barnstable County, Massachusetts, July 2021." Morbidity and Mortality Weekly Report 70, no. 30 (2021): 1059–62.

Canetti, M., N. Barda, M. Gilboa et al. "Six-Month Follow-Up After a Fourth BNT162b2 Vaccine Dose." New England Journal of Medicine 387, no. 22 (2022): 2092–94.

Chalkias, S., C. Harper, K. Vrbicky et al. "A Bivalent Omicron-Containing Booster Vaccine Against Covid-19." New England Journal of Medicine 387, no. 14 (2022): 1279–91.

Collier, A. Y., J. Miller, N. P. Hachmann et al. "Immunogenicity of the BA.5 Bivalent mRNA Vaccine Boosters." New England Journal of Medicine 388, no. 6 (2023): 565–67.

Diamond, D. "Disease Experts Warn White House of Potential for Omicron-Like Wave of Illness." Washington Post, May 5, 2023.

Goel, R. R., M. M. Painter, S. A. Apostolidis et al. "mRNA Vaccination Induces Durable Immune Memory to SARS-CoV-2 with Continued Evolution to Variants of Concern." bioRxiv, August 23, 2021. doi.org/10.1101/2021.08.23.457229.

Ladhani, S. N., G. Amirthalingam, and A. Khalil. "More on Omicron Infections in Children." New England Journal of Medicine 387, no. 20 (2022): 1911.

Lee, I. Y., C. A. Cosgrove, P. Moore et al. "A Randomized Trial Comparing Omicron-Containing Boosters With the Original Covid-19 Vaccine mRNA-1273." doi.org/10.1101/2023.01.24.23284869.

Liu, L., S. Iketani, Y. Guo et al. "Striking Antibody Evasion Manifested by the Omicron Variant of SARS-CoV-2." *Nature* 602 (2022): 676–681.

Offit, P. A. "Bivalent Covid-19 Vaccines—A Cautionary Tale." *New England Journal of Medicine* 388 (2023): 481–83.

Puranik, A., P. J. Lenehan, E. Silvert et al. "Comparison of Two Highly-Effective mRNA Vaccines for Covid-19 During Periods of Alpha and Delta Variant Prevalence." medRxiv, August 21, 2021. doi.org/10.1101/2021.08.06.21261707.

Sette, A., and S. Crotty. "Immunological Memory to SARS-CoV-2 Infection and Covid-19 Vaccines." *Immunological Reviews* 310, no. 1 (2022): 27–46.

Surie, D., J. DeCuir, Y. Zhu et al. "Early Estimates of Bivalent mRNA Vaccine Effectiveness in Preventing Covid-19-Associated Hospitalization Among Immunocompetent Adults Aged ≥65 Years—IVY Network, 18 states, September 8–November 30, 2022." *Morbidity and Mortality Weekly Report* 71, no. 5152 (2022):1625–30.

Tartof, S. Y., J. M. Slezak, H. Fischer et al. "Effectiveness of mRNA BNT162b2 Covid-19 Vaccine Up to 6 Months in a Large Integrated Health System in the USA: A Retrospective Cohort Study." *Lancet* 398, no. 10309 (2021): 1407–16.

Tartof, S. Y., J. M. Slezak, L. Puzniak et al. "Immunocompromise and Durability of BNT162b2 Vaccine Against Severe Outcomes Due to Omicron and Delta Variants." *Lancet* 10, no. 7 (2022): e61–e62.

Tenforde, M. W., W. H. Self, Y. Zhu et al. "Protection of Messenger RNA Vaccines Against Hospitalized Coronavirus Disease 2019 in Adults Over the First Year Following Authorization in the United States." *Clinical Infectious Diseases* 76, no. 3 (2023): e460–e468. doi.org/10.1093/cid/ciac381.

Wang, Q., A. Bowen, R. Valdez et al. "Antibody Response to Omicron BA.4-BA.5 Bivalent Booster." *New England Journal of Medicine* 388, no. 6 (2023): 567–69.

Yek, C., S. Warner, J. L. Wiltz et al. "Risk Factors for Severe Covid-19 Outcomes Among Persons Aged ≥18 Years Who Completed a Primary Covid-19 Vaccination Series—465 Health Care Facilities, United States, December 2020–October 2021." *Morbidity and Mortality Weekly Report* 71, no. 1 (2022): 19–25.

CHAPTER 9: TREATING COVID

Alimohamadi, Y., H. H. Tola, A. Abbasi-Ghahramanloo, et al. "Case Fatality Rate of Covid-19: A Systematic Review and Meta-Analysis." *Journal of Preventive Medicine and Hygiene* 62, no. 2 (2021): E311–E320.

Bradley, M. C., S. Perez-Vilar, Y. Chillarige et al. "Systemic Corticosteroid Use for Covid-19 in US Outpatient Settings from April 2020 to August 2021." *Journal of the American Medical Association* 327, no. 20 (2022): 2015–18.

Butler, C. C., F. D. R. Hobbs, O. A. Gbinigie et al. "Molnupiravir Plus Usual Care Versus Usual Care Alone As Early Treatment for Adults with Covid-19 at Increased Risk of Adverse Outcomes (PANORAMIC): An Open-Label, Platform-Adaptive Randomised Controlled Trial." *Lancet* 401, no. 10373 (2023). doi.org/10.1016/S0140-6736(22)02597-1.

Cao, Z., W. Gao, H. Bao et al. "VV116 Versus Nirmatrelvir-Ritonavir for Oral Treatment of Covid-19." *New England Journal of Medicine* 388, no. 5 (2022): 406–17.

Lim, S. C. L., C. P. Hor, J. H. Tay et al. "Efficacy of Ivermectin Treatment on Disease Progression Among Adults with Mild to Moderate Covid-19 and Comorbidities: The I-Tech Randomized Clinical Trial." *Journal of the American Medical Association Internal Medicine* 182, no. 4 (2022): 426–35.

Naggie, S., D. R. Boulware, C. J. Lindsell et al. "Effect of Higher-Dose Ivermectin for 6 Days vs Placebo on Time to Sustained Recovery in Outpatients with Covid-19: A Randomized Clinical Trial." *Journal of the American Medical Association* 329, no. 11 (2023): 888–97.

National Institutes of Health. "Coronavirus Disease 2019 (Covid-19) Treatment Guidelines." covid19treatmentguidelines.nih.gov (downloaded on July 18, 2022).

Pandit, J. A., J. M. Radin, D. Chiang et al. "The Paxlovid Rebound Study: A Prospective Cohort Study to Evaluate Viral and Symptom Rebound Differences Between Paxlovid and Untreated Covid-19 Participants." medRxiv, November 15, 2022. doi.org/10.1101/2022.11.14.22282195.

Planas, D., T. Bruel, I. Staropoli et al. "Resistance of Omicron Subvariants BA.2.75.2, BA.4.6, and BQ.1.1 to Neutralizing Antibodies." bioRxiv, November 17, 2022. doi.org/10.1101/2022.11.17.516888.

Reis, G., E. A. S. M. Silva, D. C. M. Silva et al. "Effect of Early Treatment with Ivermectin Among Patients with Covid-19." *New England Journal of Medicine* 386, no. 18 (2022): 1721–31.

Schmidt, P. K. Narayan, Y. Li et al. "Antibody-Mediated Protection Against Symptomatic Covid-19 Can Be Achieved at Low Serum Neutralizing Titers." *Science Translational Medicine*, March 22, 2023.

Service, R. F. "Bad News for Paxlovid? Resistance May Be Coming." *Science* (2022) 377, no. 6602: 138–39.

Shear, M. D. "Biden Tests Positive for Virus and Is Experiencing Mild Symptoms." *New York Times,* July 21, 2022.

Smith, Z. S. "The Strange Return of Ivermectin and Hydroxychloroquine: Republicans Push Drugs in State Bills." *Forbes,* May 3, 2022.

Sullivan, D. J., K. A. Gebo, S. Shoham et al. "Early Outpatient Treatment for Covid-19 with Convalescent Plasma." *New England Journal of Medicine* 386, no. 18 (2022): 1700–1711.

Tsay, S. V., M. Bartoces, K. Gouin et al. "Antibiotic Prescriptions Associated with Covid-19 Outpatient Visits Among Medicare Beneficiaries, April 2020 to April 2021." *Journal of the American Medical Association* 327, no. 20 (2022): 2018–19.

Weiland, N., M. Haberman, M. Mazzetti, and A. Karni. "Trump Was Sicker than Acknowledged with Covid-19." *New York Times,* February 11, 2021.

CHAPTER 10: LONG COVID: WHAT IS IT? CAN IT BE TREATED? CAN IT BE PREVENTED?

Akbarialiabad, H., M. H. Taghrir, A. Abdollahi et al. "Long Covid, a Comprehensive Systematic Scoping Review." *Infection* 49, no. 6 (2021): 1163–86.

Al-Aly, Z., B. Bowe, and Y. Xie. "Long Covid After Breakthrough SARS-CoV-2 Infection." *Nature Medicine* 28, no. 7 (2022): 1461–67.

Ali, S. T., A. K. Kang, T. R. Patel et al. "Evolution of Neurologic Symptoms in Non-Hospitalized Covid-19 'Long Haulers.'" *Annals of Clinical and Translational Neurology* 9, no. 7 (2022): 950–61.

Antonelli, M., R. S. Penfold, J. Merino et al. "Risk Factors and Disease Profile of Post-Vaccination SARS-CoV-2 Infection in UK Users of the Covid Symptom Study App: A Prospective, Community-Based, Nested, Case-Control Study." *Lancet* 22, no. 1 (2022): 43–55.

Antonelli, M., J. C. Pujol, T. D. Spector et al. "Risk of Long Covid Associated with Delta Versus Omicron Variants of SARS-CoV-2." *Lancet* 399, no. 10343 (2022): 2263–64.

Azzolini, E., R. Levi, R. Sarti et al. "Association Between BNT162b2 Vaccination and Long Covid After Infections Not Requiring Hospitalization in Health Care Workers." *Journal of the American Medical Association* 328, no. 7 (2022): 676–78.

Ballering, A. W., S. K. van Zon, T. C. Hartman et al. "Persistence of Somatic Symptoms After Covid-19 in the Netherlands: An Observational Cohort Study." *Lancet* 400, no. 10350 (2022): 452–61.

Barrett, C. E., A. K. Koyama, P. Alvarez et al. "Risk for Newly Diagnosed Diabetes >30 Days After SARS-CoV-2 Infection Among Persons Aged <18 Years— United States, March 1, 2020–June 28, 2021." *Morbidity and Mortality Weekly Report* 71, no. 2 (2022): 59–65.

Bonilla, H., T. C. Quach, A. Tiwari et al. "Myalgic Encephalomyelitis/Chronic Fatigue Syndrome (ME/CFS) Is Common in Post-Acute Sequelae of SARS-CoV-2 Infection (PASC): Results from a Post-Covid-19 Multidisciplinary Clinic." medRxiv, August 4, 2022. doi.org/10.1101/2022.08.03.22278363.

Brightling, C. E., and R. A. Evans. "Long Covid: Which Symptoms Can Be Attributed to SARS-CoV-2 Infection." *Lancet* 400, no. 10350 (2022): 411–13.

Buonsenso, D., D. Di Giuda, L. Sigfrid et al. "Evidence of Lung Perfusion Defects and Ongoing Inflammation in an Adolescent with Post-Acute Sequelae of SARS-CoV-2 Infection." *Lancet* 5, no. 9 (2021): 677–80.

Brown, K., A. Yahyouche, S. Haroon et al. "Long Covid and Self-Management." *Lancet* 399, no. 10322 (2022): 355.

Cachón-Zagalaz, M. Sánchez-Zafra, D. Sanabrias-Moreno et al. "Systematic Review of the Literature About the Effects of the Covid-19 Pandemic on the Lives of School Children." *Frontiers in Psychology* 11 (2020): 569348.

Canas, D., E. Molteni, J. Deng et al. "Profiling Post-Covid Syndrome Across Different Variants of SARS-CoV-2." medRxiv, July 31, 2022. doi.org/10.1101/2022.07.28.22278159.

Cha, A. E. "Vaccines May Not Prevent Many Symptoms of Long Covid, Study Suggests." *Washington Post,* May 25, 2022.

Chen, A. K., X. Wang, L. P, McCluskey et al. "Neuropsychiatric Sequelae of Long Covid-19: Pilot Results from the Covid-19 Neurological and Molecular Prospective Cohort Study in Georgia, USA." *Brain, Behavior, & Immunity* 24 (2022): 100491.

Chertow, D., S. Stein, S. Ramelli et al. "SARS-CoV-2 Infection and Persistence Throughout the Human Body and Brain." *Research Square,* December 14, 2022. doi.org/10.21203/rs.3.rs-1139035/v1.

Christensen, J. "'The Next Public Health Disaster in the Making': Studies Offer New Pieces of Long Covid Puzzle." CNN Health, August 5, 2022.

Couzin-Frankel, J. "Clues to Long Covid." *Science* 376, no. 6599 (2022).

Couzin-Frankel, J. "New Long Covid Cases Decline with Omicron." *Science* 379, no. 6638 (2023): 1174–75.

Crook, S., S. Raza, J. Nowell et al. "Long Covid-Mechanisms, Risk Factors, and Management." *British Medical Journal* 374 (2021): n1648.

Davis, H. E., G. S. Assaf, L. McCorkell et al. "Characterizing Long Covid in an International Cohort: 7 Months of Symptoms and Their Impact." *EClinicalMedicine* 38 (2021): 101019.

Devine, J. "The Dubious Origins of Long Covid." *Wall Street Journal,* March 22, 2021.

Fernandez-Castaneda, A., P. Lu, A. C. Geraghty et al. "Mild Respiratory SARS-CoV-2 Infection Can Cause Multi-Lineage Cellular Dysregulation and Myelin Loss in the Brain." bioRxiv, January 10, 2022. doi.org/10.1101/2022.01.07.475453.

Florencio, L., and C. Fernández-de-las-Penas. "Long Covid: Systemic Inflammation and Obesity As Therapeutic Targets." *Lancet Respiratory Medicine* 10, no. 8 (2022): 726–27.

Funk, A. L., N. Kupperman, T. A. Florin et al. "Post-Covid-19 Conditions Among Children 90 Days After SARS-CoV-2 Infection." *JAMA Network Open* 5, no. 7 (2022): e2223253.

Gale, J. "Striking Drop in Stress Hormone Predicts Long Covid in Study." *Bloomberg,* August 11, 2022.

George, P. M., A. U. Wells, and R. G. Jenkins. "Pulmonary Fibrosis and Covid-19: The Potential Role for Antifibrotic Therapy." *Lancet Respiratory Medicine* 8, no. 8 (2020): 807–15.

Goldstein, A., and D. Keating. "Long-Covid Symptoms Are Less Common Now Than Earlier in the Pandemic." *Washington Post,* March 18, 2023.

Gorna, R., N. MacDermott, C. Rayner et al. "Long Covid Guidelines Need to Reflect Lived Experience." *Lancet* 397, no. 10273 (2021): 455–57.

Kamrath, C., J. Rosenbauer, A. J. Eckert et al. "Incidence of Type 1 Diabetes in Children and Adolescents During the Covid-19 Pandemic in Germany: Results from the DPV Registry." *Diabetes Care* 45, no. 8 (2022): 1762–71.

Kompaniyets, L., L. Bull-Otterson, T. K. Boehmer et al. "Post-Covid-19 Symptoms and Conditions Among Children and Adolescents—United States, March 1, 2020–January 31, 2022." *Morbidity and Mortality Weekly Report* 71, no. 31 (2022): 993–99.

Lopez-Leon, S., T. Wegman-Ostrosky, N. C. A. del Valle et al. "Long-Covid in Children and Adolescents: A Systematic Review and Meta-Analyses." *Scientific Reports* 12, no. 1 (2022): 9950.

Lopilato, J. "CDC: More Clots, Kidney Failure in Kids After Covid." MedPageToday, August 5, 2022.

Mahase, E. "Covid-19: What Do We Know About 'Long Covid'?" *British Medical Journal* 370 (2020): m2815.

Mann, D. "Pandemic Brought More Woes for Kids Prone to Headaches." HealthDay, August 9, 2022.

Mariani, Mike. "The Great Gaslighting: How Covid Longhaulers Are Still Fighting for Recognition." *The Guardian,* February 3, 2022.

McNamara, D. "Long Covid Doubles Risk of Some Serious Outcomes in Children, Teens: Study." *Pediatric News,* August 5, 2022.

Mehandru, S., and M. Merad. "Pathological Sequelae of Long-Haul Covid." *Nature Immunology* 23, no. 2 (2022): 194–202.

Michelen, M., L. Manoharan, N. Elkheir et al. "Characterising Long Covid: A Living Systematic Review." *BMJ Global Health* 6, no. 9 (2021): e005427.

Nabavi, N. "Long Covid: How to Define It and How to Manage It." *British Medical Journal* 370 (2020): m3489.

Nasserie, T., M. Hittle, S. N. Goodman. "Assessment of the Frequency and Variety of Persistent Symptoms Among Patients with Covid-19: A Systematic Review." *JAMA Network Open* 4, no. 5 (2021): e2111417.

Nehme, M., P. Vetter, F. Chappuis et al. "Prevalence of Post-Coronavirus Disease Condition 12 Weeks After Omicron Infection Compared with Negative Controls and Association with Vaccination Status." *Clinical Infectious Diseases* 76, no. 9 (2022):1567–75. doi.org/10.1093/cid/ciac947.

Nittas, V., M. Gao, E. A. West et al. "Long Covid Through a Public Health Lens: An Umbrella Review." *Public Health Reviews* 43 (2022): 1604501.

O'Rourke, M. "Willed Helplessness Is the American Condition." *The Atlantic,* August 4, 2022.

Payne, D. "'Left to Rot': The Lonely Plight of Long Covid Sufferers." *Politico,* August 14, 2022.

Parasher, A. "Covid-19: Current Understanding of its Pathophysiology, Clinical Presentation and Treatment." *Postgraduate Medical Journal* 97, no. 1147 (2021): 312–20.

Phetsouphanh, C., D. R. Darley, D. B. Wilson et al. "Immunological Dysfunction Persists for 8

Months Following Initial Mild-To-Moderate SARS-CoV-2 Infection." *Nature Immunology* 23, no. 2 (2022): 210–16.

Pretorius, E., M. Vlok, C. Venter et al. "Persistent Clotting Protein Pathology in Long Covid/Post-Acute Sequelae of Covid-19 (PASC) Is Accompanied by Increased Levels of Antiplasmin." *Cardiovascular Diabetology* 20, no. 1 (2021): 172.

Rajkumar, R. P. "Covid-19 and Mental Health: A Review of the Existing Literature." *Asian Journal of Psychiatry* 52 (2020): 102066. doi.org/10.1016/j.ajp.2020.102066.

Rando, H. M., T. D. Bennett, J. B. Byrd et al. "Challenges in Defining Long Covid: Striking Differences Across Literature, Electronic Health Records, and Patient-Reported Information." medRxiv, March 26, 2021. doi.org/10.1101/2021.03.20.21253896.

Sheehan, H. "Queensland Researchers Find Overlap in Pathology of Long Covid and Chronic Fatigue Syndrome." ABC Gold Coast News, August 10, 2022.

Shulman, R., E. Cohen, T. A. Stukel, et al. "Examination of Trends in Diabetes Incidence Among Children During the Covid-19 Pandemic in Ontario, Canada, from March 2020 to September 2021." *JAMA Network Open* 5, no. 7 (2022): e2223394.

Sneller, M. C., C. J. Liang, A. R. Marques et al. "A Longitudinal Study of Covid-19 Sequelae and Immunity: Baseline Findings." *Annals of Internal Medicine* 175, no. 7 (2022): 969–79. doi.org/10.7326/M21-4905.

Su, Y., D. Yuan, D. G. Chen et al. "Multiple Early Factors Anticipate Post-Acute Covid-19 Sequelae." *Cell* 185, no. 5 (2022): 881–95.

Sudre, C. H., B. Murray, T. Varsavsky et al. "Attributes and Predictors of Long Covid." *Nature Medicine* 27, no. 4 (2021): 626–31.

Sutherland, S. "Long Covid Now Looks Like a Neurological Disease, Helping Doctors to Focus Treatments." *Scientific American* 328 (2023): 26–33.

Taquet, M., Q. Dercon, and P. J. Harrison. "Six-Month Sequelae of Post-Vaccination SARS-CoV-2 Infection: A Retrospective Cohort Study of 10,024 Breakthrough Infections." *Brain, Behavior, and Immunity* 103 (2022): 154–62.

Taquet, M., Q. Dercon, S. Luciano et al. "Incidence, Co-Occurrence, and Evolution of Long-Covid Features: A 6-Month Retrospective Cohort Study of 273,618 Survivors of Covid-19." *PLOS Med* 18, no. 9 (2021): e1003773.

Taquet, M., R. Sillett, L. Zhu et al. "Neurological and Psychiatric Risk Trajectories After SARS-CoV-2 Infection: An Analysis of 2-Year Retrospective Cohort Studies Including 1,284,437 Patients." *Lancet Psychiatry* 9, no. 10 (2022): 815–27.

Vinetz, J. "What Are the Long-Term Effects of Covid-19." *Medical News Today,* September 29, 2020.

Willan, J., G. Agarwal, and N. Bienz. "Mortality and Burden of Post-Covid-19 Syndrome Have Reduced with Time Across SARS-CoV-2 Variants in Haematology Patients." *British Journal of Haematology* 201, no. 4 (2023): 640–44.

Wisk, L. E., M. A. Gottlieb, E. S. Spatz et al. "Association of Initial SARS-CoV-2 Test Positivity with Patient-Reported Well-Being 3 Months after a Symptomatic Illness." *JAMA Network Open* 5, no. 12 (2022): e2244486.

Ziauddeen, N., D. Gurdasani, M. E. O'Hara et al. "Characteristics and Impact of Long Covid: Findings from an Online Survey." *PLOS One* 17, no. 3 (2022): e0264331.

Zollner, A., R. Koch, A. Jukic et al. "Postacute Covid-19 Is Characterized by Gut Viral Antigen Persistence in Inflammatory Bowel Diseases." *Gastroenterology* 163, no. 2 (2022): 495–506.

CHAPTER 11: CAN WE MAKE A BETTER COVID VACCINE?

INTRANASAL VACCINES

Alu, A., L. Chen, H. Tian, and X. Wei. "Intranasal Covid-19 Vaccines: From Bench to Bed." *eBioMedicine* 76 (2022): 103841. doi.org/10.1016/j.ebiom.2022.103841.

Annas, S., and M. Zamri-Saad. "Intranasal Vaccination Strategy to Control the Covid-19 Pandemic from a Veterinary Medicine Perspective." *Animals* 11 (2021): 1876. doi.org/10.3390/ani11071876.

Bastian, H. "Next Generation Covid Vaccine Update: Intranasal & Other Mucosal Vaxes." *PLOS Blogs,* July 31, 2022.

Beavis, A. C., Z. Li, K. Briggs et al. "Efficacy of Parainfluenza Virus 5 (PIV5)-Vectored Intranasal Covid-19 Vaccine as a Single Dose Vaccine and as a Booster Against SARS-CoV-2 Variants." bioRxiv, June 8, 2022. doi.org/10.1101/2022.06.07.495215.

Choudhary, O. P., Priyanka, T. A. Mohammed, and I. Singh. "Intranasal Covid-19 Vaccines: Is It a Boon or Bane?" *International Journal of Surgery* 94 (2021): 106119.

Devlin, H. "Scientists Hope Nasal Vaccines Will Help Halt Covid Transmission." *The Guardian,* August 20, 2022.

Dhama, K., M. Dhawan, R. Tiwari et al. "Covid-19 Intranasal Vaccines: Current Progress, Advantages, Prospects, and Challenges." *Human Vaccines & Immunotherapeutics* 18, no. 5 (2022): 2045853.

Diamond, D. "White House Launching $5 Billion Program to Speed Coronavirus Vaccines." *Washington Post,* April 10, 2023.

Forman, R. "Nasal Vaccination May Protect Against Respiratory Viruses Better than Injected Vaccines." Yale School of Medicine Press Release, December 21, 2021.

Hartwell, B. L., M. B. Melo, P. Xiao et al. "Intranasal Vaccination with Lipid-Conjugated Immunogens Promotes Antigen Transmucosal Uptake to Drive Mucosal and Systemic Immunity." *Science Translational Medicine* 14, no. 654 (2022): eabn1413. doi.org/10.1126/scitranslmed.abn1413.

Iwasaki, A. "Nasal Spray Booster Keeps Covid-19 at Bay." Howard Hughes Medical Institute, February 8, 2022.

Lovelace, B., Jr. "Nasal Vaccines: What's the Latest Research on Nasal Vaccines for Covid?" Yahoo! News, July 19, 2022.

Moa, T., B. Israelow, A. Suberi et al. "Unadjuvanted Intranasal Spike Vaccine Booster Elicits Robust Protective Mucosal Immunity Against Sarbecoviruses." bioRxiv, January 26, 2022. doi.org /10.1101/2022.01.24.477597.

Nalbantoglu, S. "New Nasal Vaccine Could Provide Protection Against Covid-19 Infection, Yale Study Suggests." *Yale News,* February 11, 2022.

Satija, B. "WHO Recommends New Covid Shots Should Target Only XBB Variants." Reuters, May 19, 2023.

Sridhar, G. N. "Intranasal Vax Can Bring a 'Big Positive Shift' in Fight Against Covid: Experts." *Hindu Business Line,* August 22, 2022.

Stark, F. C., B. Akache, L. Deschatelets et al. "Intranasal Immunization with a Proteosome-Adjuvanted SARS-CoV-2 Spike Protein-Based Vaccine Is Immunogenic and Efficacious in Mice and Hamsters." *Scientific Reports* 12, no. 1 (2022): 9772.

Thacker, T. "NTAGI May Soon Review Efficacy Data on India's First Intranasal Covid Vaccine." *The Economic Times,* June 2, 2022.

Topol, E., and A. Iwasaki. "Operation Nasal Vaccine— Lightning Speed to Counter Covid-19." *Science Immunology,* July 21, 2022.

van der Ley, P. A., A. Zariri, E. van Reit et al. "An Intranasal OMV-Based Vaccine Induces High Mucosal and Systemic Protecting Immunity Against a SARS-CoV-2 Infection." *Frontiers in Immunology* 12 (2021): 781280.

van Doremalen, N., J. N. Purushotham, J. E. Schulz et al. "Intranasal ChAdOx1 nCoV-19/AZD1222 Vaccination Reduces Viral Shedding After SARS-CoV-2 D614G Challenge in Preclinical Models." *Science Translational Medicine* (2021) 13, no. 607: eabh0755.

Young, K. D. "Scientists Aim to Fight Covid with Nasal Vaccine." WebMD, July 27, 2022.

PAN-SARBECOVIRUS VACCINES

Coleon, S., A. Wiedemann, M. Surénaud et al. "Design, Immunogenicity, and Efficacy of a Pan-Sarbecovirus Dendritic-Cell Targeting Vaccine." *eBioMedicine* 80 (2022): 104062.

Hurlburt, N. K., L. J. Homad, I. Sinha et al. "Structural Definition of a Pan-Sarbecovirus Neutralizing Epitope on the Spike S2 Subunit." *Communications Biology* 5, no. 11 (2022). doi.org/10.1038/ s42003-022-03262-7.

Joyce, M. G., W.-H. Chen, R. S. Sankhala et al. "SARS-CoV-2 Ferritin Nanoparticle Vaccines Elicit Broad SARS Coronavirus Immunogenicity." *Cell Reports* 37, no. 12 (2021): 110143.

Liu, Z., J. Zhou, W. Xu et al. "A Novel STING Agonist-Adjuvanted Pan-Sarbecovirus Vaccine Elicits Potent and Durable Neutralizing Antibody and T cell Responses in Mice, Rabbits, and NHPs." *Cell Research* 32 (2022): 269–87.

Martinez, D. R., A. Schäfer, S. R. Leist et al. "Chimeric Spike mRNA Vaccines Protect Against Sarbecovirus Challenge in Mice." *Science* 373, no. 6558 (2021): 991–98.

Tan, C.-W., W.-N. Chia, B. E. Young et al. "Pan-Sarbecovirus Neutralizing Antibodies in BNT162b2-Immunized SARS-CoV-1 Survivors." *New England Journal of Medicine* 385 (2021): 1401–06.

Tortorici, M. A., N. Czudnochowski, T. N. Starr et al. "Broad Sarbecovirus Neutralization by a Human Monoclonal Antibody." *Nature* 597, no. 7874 (2021): 103–108.

CHAPTER 12: SHOULD COVID VACCINES BE MANDATED?

Attkisson, S. "Republicans Seek to Combat Covid-19 Vaccine Mandate in D.C. Schools." *Sharyl Attkisson* (blog), September 21, 2022.

Bardosh, K., A. de Figueiredo, R. Gur-Arie et al. "The Unintended Consequences of Covid-19 Vaccine Policy: Why Mandates, Passports and Restrictions May Cause More Harm Than Good." *British Medical Journal Global Health* 7, no. 5 (2022): e008684. doi.org/10.1136/bmjgh-2022-008684.

Beam, A. "California Delays Coronavirus Vaccine Mandate for Schools." CNBC, April 15, 2022.

Selected Bibliography

Beard, M. "Just a Few School Districts Are Imposing Coronavirus Vaccine Mandates." *Washington Post,* August 25, 2022.

Benatar, O. "Columbus Measles Cases Rise to 32." NBC4, November 28, 2022.

"Canada to Lift Covid Vaccine Requirement for Travelers at Border." *Detroit News,* September 21, 2022.

Charles, J. "Breaking: Judge Strikes Down Federal Mask and Vaccine Mandate in Schools." *RedState,* September 21, 2022.

Colton, E. "McCarthy Vows Military Vaccine Mandate Will End or National Defense Bill Won't Move Forward." FoxNews.com, December 4, 2022.

Copp, T. "Keep Covid-19 Military Vaccine Mandate, Defense Secretary Says." *Military Times,* December 4, 2022.

Cropley, J. "HVCC Reinstates Covid Vaccination Mandate for Fall Semester." *The Daily Gazette,* August 22, 2022.

Daniels, N. "Should Schools Require Students to Get the Coronavirus Vaccine?" *New York Times,* September 15, 2021.

"Federal Court Ruling Tosses Lawsuit, Keeps Michigan State University's Covid Vaccine Mandate." WILX 10, February 23, 2022.

"Federal Court Sides with New York in Fight Over School Vaccine Rules." Associated Press, July 29, 2022.

Freking, K. "Senate Passes Defense Bill Rescinding Covid-19 Vaccine Mandate." Associated Press, December 15, 2022.

Goddard, K., J. G. Donohue, N. Lewis et al. "Safety of Covid-19 mRNA Vaccination Among Young Children in the Vaccine Safety Datalink." *Pediatrics* 152, no, 1 (2023): e2023061894.

Harvard University Health Services. "Covid-19 Vaccine Requirement." January 2021. huhs.harvard.edu/covid-19-vaccine-requirement-faqs.

Hoffman, J. "Opposition to School Vaccine Mandates Has Grown Significantly, Study Finds." *New York Times,* December 16, 2022.

Hogan, B., and S. Algar. "Gov. Hochul Wants a School Vaccine Mandate Before Fall 2022 Semester." *New York Post,* December 17, 2021.

Howard, J. "More States Are Banning Covid-19 Vaccine Mandates in Schools. Here Are the Shots Already Required." NBC5, July 21, 2021.

Hui, K. "Will Covid-19 Vaccines Be Required in Schools?" VeryWell Health, July 22, 2021.

Issa, N. "CPS Employee Vaccine Mandate Reinstated by Illinois Appellate Court." *Chicago Sun Times,* April 21, 2022.

Jindal, B., and H. Overton. "You Can Oppose School Covid-Vaccine Mandates Without Opposing Vaccines." *National Review,* March 15, 2022.

Kamenetz, A. "Should Schools Require the Covid Vaccine? Many Experts Say It's Too Soon." NPR, November 19, 2021.

Kheel, R. "Vaccine Mandate is Hurting Recruiting, Top Marine General Says." Military.com, December 4, 2022.

Laila, C. "Trump-Appointed Judge Strikes Down Federal School Mask and Vaccine Mandate." *Gateway Pundit,* September 21, 2022.

"Mayor Adams Launches Covid-19 Booster Campaign, Announces Additional Flexibility for NYC Businesses, Parents." *NYC,* September 20, 2022.

"Military to Keep Covid Vaccine Mandate." CapRadio, December 6, 2022.

Nelson, J. Q. "Oregon Parents Petition State Health Board to End Covid Vaccine Mandates in School." *New York Post,* September 14, 2022.

"New Lawsuit Challenges End of Vaccine Mandate Exemption." Associated Press, February 24, 2022.

North, A. "Will Schools Require Covid-19 Vaccines for Students?" *Vox,* February 11, 2022.

NVIC Advocacy Team. "NVIC's 2022 Annual Report on U.S. State Vaccine Legislation." November 17, 2022. nvic.org/newsletter/nov-2022/annual-state-vaccine-legislation-report.

Parasidis, E. "Covid-19 Vaccine Mandates at the Supreme Court: Scope and Limits of Federal Authority." *Health Affairs,* March 8, 2022.

Poff, J. "Colleges Cling to Covid-19 Mask and Vaccine Mandates as School Year Begins." *Washington Examiner,* August 31, 2022.

Poff, J. "DC Schools Mandate Vaccine Doses as Other Districts Move Past Covid Restrictions." *Washington Examiner,* August 16, 2022.

Pryor, P. A. "Challenges Against Employer Covid-19 Vaccine Mandates Show No Sign of Slowing." *National Law Review,* September 19, 2022.

Romanelli, J. N. "Against Vaccine Mandates for Schoolchildren." *Wall Street Journal,* August 11, 2022.

Sequeira, K. "LAUSD School Board Delays Covid-19 Vaccine Mandate to Align with State." EdSource, May 11, 2022.

Shepardson, D. "United Airlines to Let Unvaccinated

Employees Return to Jobs March 28—Memo." *Reuters*, March 10, 2022.

Stavely, Z. "Vaccine Mandate for Schools Delayed Until at Least July 2023." *EdSource*, April 15, 2022.

Wooten, A. "Federal Judge Strikes Down Covid-19 Vaccine and Mask Mandates for Head Start Students, Teachers." *Just the News*, September 21, 2022.

CHAPTER 13: IS IMMUNITY FROM NATURAL INFECTION BETTER THAN VACCINATION?

Boyton, R. J., and D. M. Altmann. "Risk of SARS-CoV-2 Reinfection After Natural Infection." *Lancet* 397, no. 10280 (2021): 1161–63.

Brusselaers, N., D. Steadson, K. Bjorklund et al. "Evaluation of Science Advice During the Covid-19 Pandemic in Sweden." *Humanities and Social Sciences Communications* 9, no. 91 (2022). doi.org/10.1057/s41599-022-01097-5.

Carazo, S., S. M. Skowronski, M. Brisson et al. "Protection Against Omicron (B.1.1.529) BA.2 Reinfection Conferred by Primary Omicron BA.1 or Pre-Omicron SARS-CoV-2 Infection Among Health-Care Workers with and Without mRNA Vaccination: A Test-Negative Case-Control Study." *Lancet Infectious Diseases* 23, no. 1 (2023): 45–55.

Cavanaugh, A. M., K. B. Spicer, D. Thoroughman et al. "Reduced Risk of Reinfection with SARS-CoV-2 After Covid-19 Vaccination—Kentucky, May–June 2021." *Morbidity and Mortality Weekly Report* 70, no. 32 (2021): 1081–83.

Chen, Y., P. Tong, N. Whiteman et al. "Immune Recall Improves Antibody Durability and Breadth to SARS-CoV-2 Variants." *Science Immunology* 7, no. 78 (2022). doi.org/10.1126/sciimmunol.abp8328.

Covid-19 Forecasting Team. "Past SARS-CoV-2 Infection Protection Against Re-Infection: A Systematic Review and Meta-Analysis." *Lancet* 401, no. 10379 (2023): 833–42. doi.org/10.1016/S0140-6736(22)02465-5.

Gazit, S., R. Shlezinger, G. Perez et al. "Severe Acute Respiratory Syndrome Coronavirus 2 (SARS-CoV-2) Naturally Acquired Immunity versus Vaccine-induced Immunity, Reinfections versus Breakthrough Infections: A Retrospective Cohort Study." *Clinical Infectious Diseases* 75, no. 1 (2022): e545–e551.

Goldberg, Y., M. Mandel, Y. M. Bar-On et al. "Protection and Waning of Natural and Hybrid Immunity to SARS-CoV-2." *New England Journal of Medicine* 386, no. 23 (2022): 2201–12.

Goldberg, Y., M. Mandel, Y. Woodbridge et al. "Similarity of Protection Conferred by Previous SARS-CoV-2 Infection and by BNT162b2 Vaccine: A 3-Month Nationwide Experience From Israel." *American Journal of Epidemiology* 191, no. 8 (2022): 1420–28.

Hanrath, A. T., B. A. I. Payne, and C. Duncan. "Prior SARS-CoV-2 Infection Is Associated with Protection Against Symptomatic Reinfection." *Journal of Infection* 82, no. 4 (2021): e29–e30.

Hansen, C. H., D. Michlmayr, S. M. Gubbels et al. "Assessment of Protection Against Reinfection with SARS-CoV-2 Among 4 Million PCR-Tested Individuals in Denmark in 2020: A Population-Level Observational Study." *Lancet* 397, no. 10280 (2021): 1202–12.

Howard, J. "As Measles Outbreak Sickens More Than a Dozen Children in Ohio, Local Health Officials Seek Help from CDC." *CNN*, November 17, 2022.

Juul, F. E., H. C. Jodal, I. Barua et al. "Mortality in Norway and Sweden During the Covid-19 Pandemic." *Scandinavian Journal of Public Health* 50, no. 1 (2022): 38–45.

Katz, M. H. "Protection Because of Prior SARS-CoV-2 Infection." *Journal of the American Medical Association Internal Medicine* 181, no. 10 (2021): 1409.

Leidi, A., F. Koegler, R. Dumont et al. "Risk of Reinfection After Seroconversion to Severe Acute Respiratory Syndrome Coronavirus 2 (SARS-CoV-2): A Population-Based Propensity-Score Matched Cohort Study." *Clinical Infectious Diseases* 74, no. 4 (2022): 622–29.

León, T. M., V. Dorabawila, L. Nelson et al. "Covid-19 Cases and Hospitalizations by Covid-19 Vaccination Status and Previous Covid-19 Diagnosis—California and New York, May–November 2021." *Morbidity and Mortality Weekly Report* 71, no. 4 (2022): 125–31.

Lumley, S. F., D. O'Donnell, N. E. Stoesser et al. "Antibody Status and Incidence of SARS-CoV-2 Infection in Health Care Workers." *New England Journal of Medicine* 384, no. 6 (2021): 533–40.

Lumley, S. F., G. Rodger, B. Constantinides et al. "An Observational Cohort Study on the Incidence of Severe Acute Respiratory Syndrome Coronavirus 2 (SARS-CoV-2) Infection and B.1.1.7 Variant Infection in Healthcare Workers by Antibody and Vaccination Status." *Clinical Infectious Diseases* 74, no. 7 (2022): 1208–19.

Sheehan, M. M., A. J. Reddy, and M. B. Rothberg. "Reinfection Rates Among Patients Who Previously Tested Positive for Coronavirus Disease 2019: A

Retrospective Cohort Study." *Clinical Infectious Diseases* 73, no. 10 (2021): 1882–86.

Shenai, M. B., R. Rahme, and H. Noorchashm. "Equivalency of Protection from Natural Immunity in Covid-19 Recovered Versus Fully Vaccinated Persons: A Systematic Review and Pooled Analysis." *Cureus* 13, no. 10 (2021): e19102. doi.org/10.7759/cureus.19102.

Shrestha, N. K., P. C. Burke, A. S. Nowakci et al. "Necessity of Coronavirus Disease 2019 (Covid-19) Vaccination in Persons Who Have Already Had Covid-19." *Clinical Infectious Diseases* 75, no. 1 (2022): e662–e671.

Tu, W., P. Zhang, A. Roberts et al. "SARS-CoV-2 Infection, Hospitalization, and Death in Vaccinated and Infected Individuals by Age Groups in Indiana, 2021-2022." *American Journal of Public Health* 113, no. 1 (2023): 96–104.

Vitale, J., N. Mumoli, P. Clerici et al. "Assessment of SARS-CoV-2 Reinfection 1 Year After Primary Infection in a Population in Lombardy, Italy." *Journal of the American Medical Association Internal Medicine* 181, no. 10 (2021): 1407–08.

The Week Staff. "Did Sweden's Covid-19 Experiment Pay Off in the End?" *The Week*, September 8, 2022.

Wilkins, J. T., L. R. Hirschhorn, E. L. Gray et al. "Serologic Status and SARS-CoV-2 Infection Over 6 Months of Follow Up in Healthcare Workers in Chicago: A Cohort Study." *Infection Control and Hospital Epidemiology* 43, no. 9 (2022): 1207–15.

Wong, J. Y., J. K. Cheung, Y. Lin et al., "Intrinsic and Effective Severity of Covid-19 Cases Infected with the Ancestral Strain and Omicron BA.2 Variant in Hong Kong," *The Journal of Infectious Diseases* (2023) doi.org/10.1093/infdis/jiad236.

Woodbridge, Y., S. Amit, A. Huppert et al. "Viral Load Dynamics of SARS-CoV-2 Delta and Omicron Variants Following Multiple Vaccine Doses and Previous Infection." *Nature Communications* (2022) 13: 6706.

CHAPTER 14: A PRACTICAL GUIDE TO COVID TODAY

Bhattacharyya, R. P., and W. P. Hanage. "Challenges in Inferring Intrinsic Severity of the SARS-CoV-2 Omicron Variant." *New England Journal of Medicine* 386, no. 7 (2022): e14.

Brüssow, H. "Covid-19: Omicron—The Latest, the Least Virulent, But Probably Not the Last Variant of Concern of SARS-CoV-2." *Microbial Biotechnology* 15, no. 7 (2022): 1927–39.

Collier, A. Y., J. Miller, N. P. Hachmann et al. "Immunogenicity of the BA.5 Bivalent mRNA Vaccine Boosters." *New England Journal of Medicine* 388, no. 6 (2023): 565–67.

Halasa, N. B., S. M. Olson, M. A. Staat et al. "Maternal Vaccination and Risk of Hospitalization for Covid-19 Among Infants." *New England Journal of Medicine* 387, no. 2 (2022): 109–19.

Haseltine, W. A. "Omicron: Less Virulent but Still Dangerous," *Forbes*, January 11, 2022.

Hui, K. P. Y., J. C. W. Ho, M. Cheung et al. "SARS-CoV-2 Omicron Variant Replication in Human Bronchus and Lung Ex Vivo." *Nature* 603, no. 7902 (2022): 715–20.

Kurhade, C., J. Zou, H. Xia et al. "Low Neutralization of SARS-CoV-2 Omicron BA.2.75.2, BQ.1.1, and XBB.1 by Parental mRNA Vaccine or a BA.5-Bivalent Booster." *Nature Medicine* 29, no. 2 (2022): 344–47. nature.com/articles/s41591-022-02162-x.

Lewnard, J. A., V. X. Hong, M. M. Patel et al. "Clinical Outcomes Among Patients Infected with Omicron (B.1.1.529) SARS-CoV-2 Variant in Southern California." *Nature Medicine* 28 (2022): 1933–43.

Link-Gelles, R., A. A. Ciesla, K. E. Fleming-Dutra et al. "Effectiveness of Bivalent mRNA Vaccines in Preventing Symptomatic SARS-CoV-2 Infection—Increasing Community Access to Testing Program, United States, September-November 2022." *Morbidity and Mortality Weekly Report* 71, no. 48 (2022): 1526–30.

Nealon, J., and B. J. Cowling. "Omicron Severity: Milder but Not Mild." *Lancet* 399, no. 10323 (2022): 412–13.

Offit, P. A. "Bivalent Covid-19 Vaccines—A Cautionary Tale." *New England Journal of Medicine* 388, no. 6 (2023): 481–83.

Planas, D., T. Bruel, I. Staropoli et al. "Resistance of Omicron Subvariants BA.2.75.2, BA.4.6, and BQ.1.1 to Neutralizing Antibodies." bioRxiv, November 17, 2022. doi.org/10.1101/2022.11.17.516888.

Prahl, M., Y. Golan, and A. G. Cassidy. "Evaluation of Transplacental Transfer of mRNA Vaccine Products and Functional Antibodies During Pregnancy and Infancy." *Nature Communications* 13, no. 1 (2022): 4422. doi.org/10.1038/S41467-022-32188-1.

Satija, B. "WHO Recommends New Covid Shots Should Target Only XBB Variants." Reuters, May 19, 2023.

Shimabukuro, T. T., S. Y. Kim, T. R. Myers et al. "Preliminary Findings of mRNA Covid-19 Vaccine Safety in Pregnant Persons." *New England Journal of Medicine* 384, no. 24 (2021): 2273–82.

Surie, D., J. DeCuir, Y. Zhu et al. "Early Estimates of Bivalent mRNA Vaccine Effectiveness in Preventing Covid-19-Associated Hospitalization Among Immunocompetent Adults Aged ≥65 Years—IVY Network, 18 States, September 8–November 30, 2022." *Morbidity and Mortality Weekly Report* 71, no. 5152 (2022): 1625–30.

Tenforde, M. W., Z. A. Weber, K. Natarajan et al. "Early Estimates of Bivalent mRNA Vaccine Effectiveness in Preventing Covid-19-Associated Emergency Department or Urgent Care Encounters and Hospitalizations Among Immunocompetent Adults—VISION Network, Nine States, September–November 2022." *Morbidity and Mortality Weekly Report* 71, no. 5152 (2022): 1616–24.

Wang, L., N. A. Berger, D. C. Kaelber et al. "Comparison of Outcomes from Covid Infection in Pediatric and Adult Patients Before and After the Emergence of Omicron." medRxiv, January 2, 2022. doi.org/10.1101/2021.12.30.21268495.

Wang, Q., A. Bowen, R. Valdez et al. "Antibody Responses to Omicron BA.4/BA.5 Bivalent mRNA Vaccine Booster Shot." *New England Journal of Medicine* 388 (2023): 567–69.

Xie, Y., T. Choi, and Z. Al-Aly. "Nirmatrelvir and the Risk of Post-Acute Sequelae of Covid-19." medRxiv, November 5, 2022. doi.org/10.1101/2022.11.03.22281783.

EPILOGUE: LESSONS LEARNED (OR NOT)

Gutman-Wei, R. "Inside the Mind of an Anti-Paxxer." *The Atlantic*, November 22, 2022.

Klann, J. G., Z. H. Strasser, M. R. Hutch et al. "Distinguishing Admissions Specifically for Covid-19 from Incidental SARS-CoV-2 Admissions: National Retrospective Electronic Health Record Study." *Journal of Medical Internet Research* 24, no. 5 (2022): e37931.

Mast, J. "Infectious Disease Board Recommends Hospitals Stop Screening Asymptomatic Patients for Covid-19." *STAT*, December 21, 2022.

News Service of Florida. "The Florida Supreme Court Impanels a Grand Jury to Investigate Covid Vaccines." WFSU, December 22, 2022.

Tayag, Y. "How Many Republicans Died Because the GOP Turned Against Vaccines?" *The Atlantic*, December 23, 2022.

Weber, L., and J. Achenbach. "Covid Backlash Hobbles Public Health and Future Pandemic Response." *Washington Post*, March 8, 2023.

INDEX

ABOUT THE AUTHOR

PAUL A. OFFIT, M.D., is the director of the Vaccine Education Center at the Children's Hospital of Philadelphia, as well as the Maurice R. Hilleman Professor of Vaccinology and a professor of pediatrics at the Perelman School of Medicine at the University of Pennsylvania. A graduate of Tufts University and the University of Maryland Medical School, he is the recipient of many awards, including the J. Edmund Bradley Prize for Excellence in Pediatrics from the University of Maryland Medical School, the Young Investigator Award in Vaccine Development from the Infectious Disease Society of America, and a Research Career Development Award from the National Institutes of Health.

Offit has published more than 180 papers in medical and scientific journals in the areas of rotavirus-specific immune responses and vaccine safety. He is also the co-inventor of the rotavirus vaccine, RotaTeq, recommended for universal use in infants by the Centers for Disease Control and Prevention in 2006 and by the World Health Organization in 2013. For this achievement, he received the Luigi Mastroianni and William Osler Awards from the University of Pennsylvania School of Medicine, the Charles Mérieux Award from the National Foundation for Infectious Diseases, and was honored by Bill and Melinda Gates during the launch of their foundation's Living Proof Project for global health.

In 2009, Offit received the President's Certificate for Outstanding Service from the American Academy of Pediatrics. In 2011, he received the David E. Rogers Award from the Association of American Medical

Colleges, the Odyssey Award from the Center for Medicine in the Public Interest, and was elected to the Institute of Medicine of the National Academy of Sciences. In 2012, Offit received the Distinguished Medical Achievement Award from the College of Physicians of Philadelphia; in 2013, he received the Maxwell Finland Award for Scientific Achievement from the National Foundation for Infectious Diseases and the Distinguished Alumnus Award from the University of Maryland School of Medicine. In 2015, Offit won the Lindback Award for Distinguished Teaching from the University of Pennsylvania and was elected to the American Academy of Arts and Sciences. In 2016, he won the Franklin Founder Award from the city of Philadelphia, the Porter Prize from the University of Pittsburgh School of Public Health, the Lifetime Achievement Award from the Philadelphia Business Journal, and the Jonathan E. Rhoads Medal for Distinguished Service to Medicine from the American Philosophical Society. In 2018, Offit received the Gold Medal from the Sabin Vaccine Institute; in 2019, the John P. McGovern Award from the American Medical Writers Association; and in 2020 the Public Educator Award from CHILD USA. In 2021, Offit was awarded the Edward Jenner Lifetime Achievement Award in Vaccinology from the 15th Vaccine Congress and was elected to the Baltimore Jewish Hall of Fame. In 2022, Offit received the Mentor of the Year Award from the Eastern Society for Pediatric Research and the Dean's Alumni Leadership Award from the University of Maryland School of Medicine. In 2023, Offit was elected to membership in the American Philosophical Society.

Formerly a member of the Advisory Committee on Immunization Practices to the Centers for Disease Control and Prevention, Offit is currently a member of the FDA's vaccine advisory committee and is a founding advisory board member of the Autism Science Foundation and the Foundation for Vaccine Research.